Antiandrogen-Estrogen Therapy for Signs of Androgenization

New Developments in Biosciences 3

New Developments in Biosciences publishes the Proceedings of scientific symposia and workshops sponsored by SCHERING AG

Important notice
Medical science is constantly developing. Research and clinical experience expand our knowledge, especially with regard to treatment and medication.

For dosages and applications mentioned in this work, the reader may rely on the authors, editors and publisher having taken great pains as to ensure that these indications reflect the standard of knowledge at the time this work was completed.

Nevertheless, every user is requested to check the package leaflet of the medication, in order to determine on one's own account whether the recommendations given for the dosages or the likely contra-indications differ from those given in this book. This is especially true for medication which is seldom used or has recently been put on the market and for medication whose application has been restricted by the German Ministry of Health.

Walter de Gruyter
Berlin · New York 1987

Antiandrogen-Estrogen Therapy for Signs of Androgenization

Editor
Adolf E. Schindler

Walter de Gruyter
Berlin · New York 1987

Editor
Prof. Dr. med. Adolf E. Schindler
Direktor
Zentrum für Frauenheilkunde
Universitätsklinikum Essen
Hufelandstrasse 55
D-4300 Essen 1

This book contains 101 illustrations and 59 tables.

Library of Congress Cataloging-in-Publication Data

Antiandrogen-estrogen therapy for signs of androgenization.
(New developments in biosciences; 3)
Proceedings of a conference.
Bibliography: p.
1. Virilism--Chemotherapy--Congresses. 2. Antiandrogens--Congresses. 3. Estrogen--Therapeutic use--Congresses. I. Schindler, A. E. (Adolf E.), 1936- . II. Title: Anti-androgen-estrogen therapy for signs of androgenization. III. Series.
RG 208.A57 1987 615'.766 87-8924
ISBN 0-89925-304-0 (U.S.)

CIP-Kurztitelaufnahme der Deutschen Bibliothek

Antiandrogen-estrogen therapy for signs of androgenization / ed. Adolf E. Schindler. -
Berlin; New York: de Gruyter, 1987.
(New developments in biosciences; 3)
ISBN 3-11-011226-4
NE: Schindler, Adolf E. [Hrsg.]; GT

Welcome address

C. Flamigni

Mr. Chairman of the Congress, Colleagues, Ladies and Gentlemen,

I have accepted with pleasure the invitation of the organizers of this Congress to extend a welcome, in my own name, if I may say so, and in that of Italian gynecologists, endocrinologists, research workers to all of you gathered here today for an International Congress on one of the most important and significant molecules in the history of endocrinological pharmacology, utilized in many areas of clinical medicine.

I was very happy to come here to deliver this welcome for a number of reasons: for the pleasure of meeting again old friends, people I had not seen for a long time, for the pleasure and curiosity of meeting famous research workers with whom I was acquainted only through their works, and owing to the long-standing as well as useful cooperation with Schering, that has been going on for a long, long time. And I must say that as usually happens to people who are past fifty, it is the evocative memory that chiefly dominates among cerebral activities: this invitation to come here and talk to you of this important progestational molecule has reminded me of a series of facts and events of my past life, back in 1968, the first time I met Dr. Neumann in Berlin where I went with a very dear friend of mine and of Schering's, a very prominent gentleman researcher, Ian Sommerville, who unfortunately is not here with us today to join me in welcoming you. And then later on in time, in 1971, at the time of a strange event which Dr. Neumann is perhaps hearing of today for the first time, the invasion of the town of Bologna by his mice.

We were carrying out research on feminized mice that Dr. Neumann sent us to Bologna by plane, but these mice got blocked at the Bologna airport by a sort of mild hysterical attack on the part of the official vet for the province who did not want these mysterious mice, affected with these shocking morphological alterations, in his town, perhaps for fear of an epidemic. During the time we were fighting to get these mice cleared through the customs, they literally ate their way through the bottom of their cage, so by the time we cleared them and collected them, they fled in all directions. Bologna is a town of great liberal traditions, so I'm quite sure that these mice have led happy, serene lives, perhaps they have even had a sex life after their escape into the town.

Something else that comes into my mind, but that is much more serious than this, is the wonderful relationship that we in our Institute of Physiopathology of Reproduction in Bologna have had for a long time with this molecule in treating hirsutism of various types. Many years ago we had already published the first 500 cases treated with cyproterone acetate at more conventional doses in association with ethinyl estradiol, and more recently we have published 550 more cases. Altogether, the number of hirsute women treated is over 1300 with a very low dropout rate as regards the treatment, equal to about 8%—9%, and with highly successful results both with regard to the treatment of hirsutism and to that of acne. We have also been able to record excellent results with associations that include the use of very low doses of ethinyl estradiol, which we use in quantities of only 20 mcg in the first two weeks and of 30 mcg in the third week, and we have been able to record satisfactory results especially when the overall duration of the therapy exceeded 3 years.

Another thing I can remember with pleasure, still with reference to these treatments, is the use of associations at low doses: Diane, until the latter association became available and now this low-dose association with a lower quantity of ethinyl estradiol. And here our experience is that success both as regards the treatment of acne and as regards the continuation of the treatment of major hirsutism as maintenance therapies, but especially in a very particular group of young women, that is to say, those that leave the stage of multifollicularity and approach the formation of micropolycystic ovaries and begin to show early signs of hyperandrogeny and hirsutism. I do not know whether these topics are going to be dealt with here, but there is a report of Professor Falsetti on the treatment of micropolycystic ovaries where these issues might appear to be relevant.

I think I have amply used up the time allotted to me for this introduction, for this welcome, a welcome I am glad to repeat and which I extend in the hope that this meeting—and I am certain my hope will be realized—prove profitable, useful, important to all of us. Thank you.

Contents

Introduction

A. A. Haspels, N. van der Vange

Update on antiandrogen-estrogen therapy: cyproterone acetate (2 mg) and ethinyl estradiol (0.035 mg)

"The life of a doctor dealing with family planning and the methods used is never dull" [4].

When the contraceptive pill was first introduced more than 25 years ago contraceptive pills had to be used in doses large enough to assure the minimization of unwanted pregnancy. Later in 1968 in the People's Republic of China, contraceptive pills with reduced doses were used with good contraceptive efficacy. These contained 0.035 mg ethinyl estradiol combined with low-dose norethisterone.

Cyproterone acetate has been widely tested for the treatment of acne and hypertrichosis. It was first used in reverse sequential therapy by Hammerstein [7] in high doses of 100 mg day with 0.050 mg of ethinyl estradiol. It was subsequently observed that a considerable lower dose of cyproterone acetate led to undoubted therapeutic success [5]. I have personally observed patients who had used tetracyclines for 10 years without much success, who were without acne after three months of cyproterone acetate use. For a long time, we have advocated a policy of changing patients from higher to lower dose pills, not for the reasons of potency, but because the low-dose pills are associated with lower metabolic and cardiovascular risk than higher-dose pills. The low-dose pills are just as good and have been readily available since 1974.

As it is clear that 2 mg cyproterone acetate is sufficient to prevent ovulation, it should be preferable to combine it with 0.035 mg ethinyl estradiol rather than with 0.050 mg of this substance. As mentioned by Aydinlik (1986) [2], in 1974 I started to use this low-dose combination which was produced in our hospital pharmacy in Utrecht with excellent results. A double-blind study with Diane-50® and Diane-35® was performed [2] in Germany, Austria, England, France, Italy, Denmark, Switzerland and Holland. As could be expected, estrogen side effects were reduced with Diane-35®: breast tension, edema, nausea, vomiting, chloasma, varicosis and weight gain. By the ninth cycle 13% of the clients using Diane-35® had a weight gain of 2 kg. The percentage for Diane-50® users was 21%.

Moreover, an interesting conclusion was that acne disappeared earlier with Diane-35® than with Diane-50®. The reason for this could be that a high dose of estradiol has a large inhibitory effect upon human adrenal 3β-hydroxysteroid dehydrogenase activity [3]. To put it simply a low dose of ethinyl estradiol results in less inhibition of 3β-HSD activity resulting in a smaller production of adrenal DHEA and DHEAS.

Sex Hormone Binding Globulin (SHBG) and Corticosteroid Binding Globulin (CGB)

The effect of an oral contraceptive on SHBG level is, as is the effect on hepatic lipase, a balance between estrogenic and androgenic properties [8]. Ethinyl estradiol induces a rise in SHBG. This rise is counteracted by the androgenic activity of progestagens.

Compared to the other six preparations, Diane-35® results in the highest SHBG values, again an expression of lack of androgenicity. Regarding CBG levels: monophasic CPA induced higher CBG values than the other six preparations, which did not differ in effect from each other (figs 1 A and 1 B, tab. 1). This also implies that, as SHBG is the carrier protein for testosterone, the bound fraction of testosterone increases, while the free, biologically active fraction decreases. This is an additional advantage besides the action of cyproterone acetate on the androgen receptor.

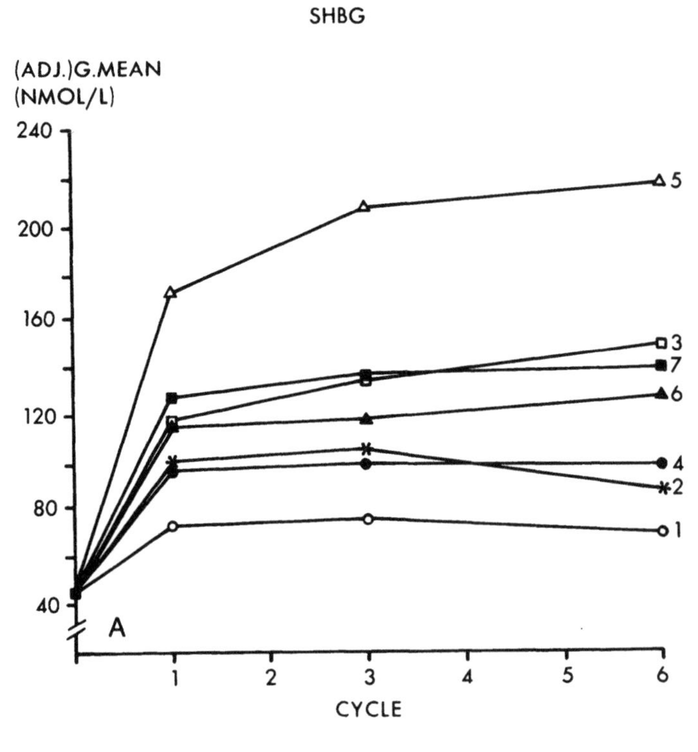

Fig. 1A

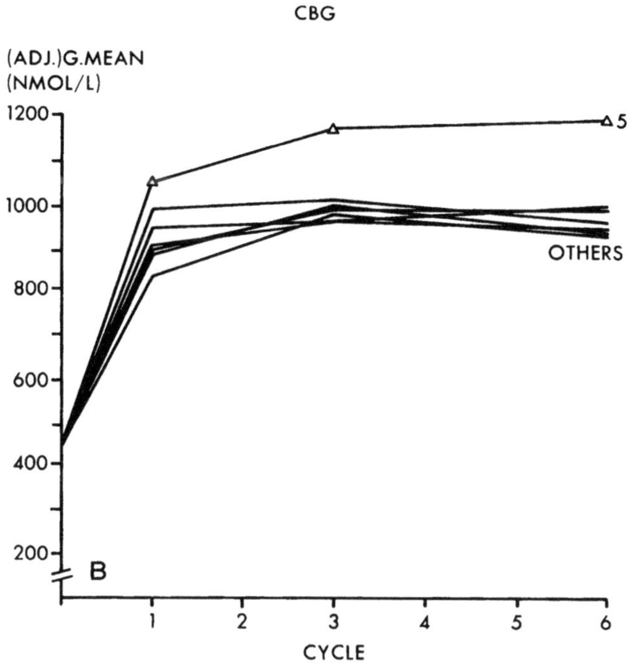

Fig. 1B

Fig. 1 Effects of monophasic LNG (.1.; o———o), monophasic NET (.2.; x———x), monophasic DSG (.3.; □———□), triphasic LNG (.4.; •———•), monophasic CPA (.5.; △———△), triphasic GSD (.6.; ▲———▲) and biphasic DSG (.7.; ■———■) on plasma levels of SHBG (A) and CBG (B) in 70 healthy women. The adjusted mean values (corrected for differences in pretreatment values) are presented.

Table 1 Oral contraceptive preparations: composition and intake regimen

Preparation	Days	Amount oft ethinyl estradiol (μg)	Amount and type of the progestagen (μg)	
1. Monophasic LNG	21	30	150	levonorgestrel
2. Monophasic NET	21	35	1000	norethisterone
3. Monophasic DSG	21	30	150	desogestrel
4. Triphasic LNG	6	30	50	levonorgestrel
	5	40	75	levonorgestrel
	10	30	125	levonorgestrel
5. Monophasic CPA	21	35	2000	cyproterone acetate
6. Triphasic GSD	6	30	50	gestoden
	5	40	70	gestoden
	10	30	100	gestoden
7. Biphasic DSG	7	40	25	desogestrel
	14	30	125	desogestrel

Lipid metabolism

Exogenous steroids affect lipid metabolism: estrogens increase HDL-cholesterol and triglycerides, whereas most progestagens increase LDL-cholesterol and decrease HDL-cholesterol. The effect of the progestagens must be attributed to their intrinsic androgenic properties and is, therefore, dose and type dependent. Epidemiologic studies [6, 8] have shown that the HDL-cholesterol particle has an inverse relationship with the incidence of cardiovascular disease, especially its subfraction HDL 2. The LDL-cholesterol level is positively associated with cardiovascular disease.

HDL-C levels are lowered by progestagens with intrinsic androgenicity, because of stimulation of hepatic lipase [9]. This enzyme is responsible for the catabolism of HDL 2. The activity of hepatic lipase is stimulated by androgens and decreased by estrogens. Therefore, the ultimate effect of a combined oral contraceptive on hepatic lipase and consequently its effect on HDL 2 will be determined by the hormonal composition of the preparations.

In our hospital we compared the effect of Diane-35® on lipid metabolism with six other low-dose oral contraceptives which had about the same amount of ethinyl estradiol (30—35 mcg), but different types and doses of progestagens (tab. 1). Except for cyproterone acetate, all other progestagens were 19-nortestosterone derivatives and thus had, in some degree, androgenic properties.

In comparison with the other preparations Diane-35® and biphasic desogestrel induced the highest HDL 2 levels (fig. 2). The highest values for total HDL-cholesterol, Apo A—I, HDL 2 cholesterol, HDL 2 phospholipids, HDL 3 cholesterol and HDL 3 phospholipids were consistently found for monophasic cyproterone acetate (fig 3). The following ranking from high to low of the intrinsic androgenicity of the progestagens has been found:

levonorgestrel > gestoden > norethisterone = 3 ketodesogestrel > cyproterone acetate.

The positive effect of ethinyl estradiol on HDL was not opposed by intrinsic androgenic activity [10].

Carbohydrate metabolism and vitamin B_6

In the same study, carbohydrate metabolism and the vitamin B_6 status were also studied. There was no adverse effect on either shortterm parameters of carbohydrate metabolism (fasting glucose and insulin levels, and glucose challenge testing) or longterm parameters (glycosylated haemoglobin (HbA_1) and glycosylated proteins) during treatment for six months with Diane-35®. The same observation was made for the vitamin B_6 status: There was no change in the erythrocyte transaminase (EGOT) level, which is an indirect parameter of vitamin B_6 and plasma pyridoxal-5′-phosphate levels during Diane-35® treatment over six months.

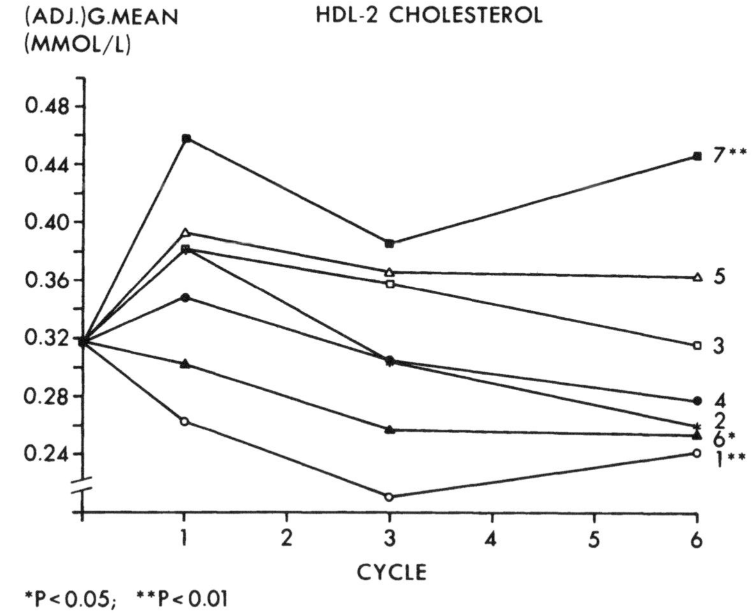

Fig. 2 Effects of the seven preparations on HDL-2 cholesterol. For explanation of the symbols see figure I.

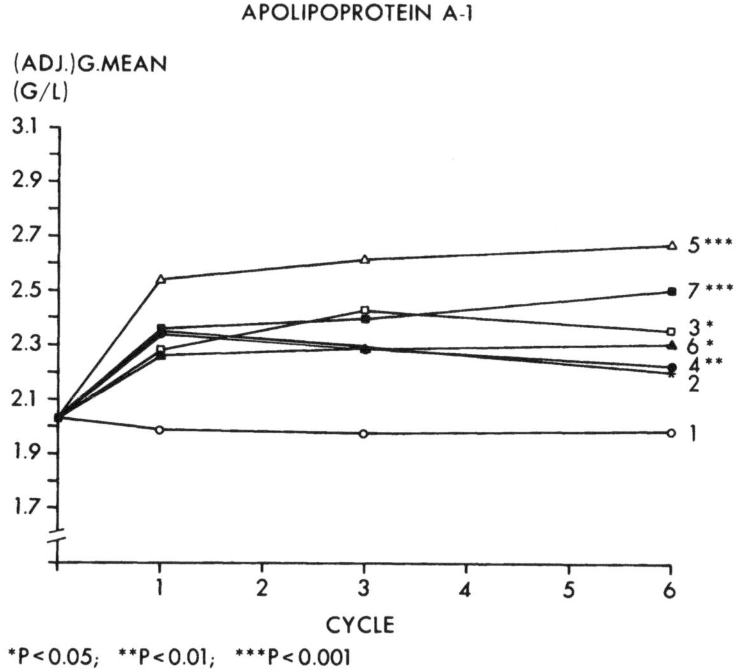

Fig. 3 Effects of the seven preparations on apolipoprotein A —I. For explanation of the symbols see figure 1.

Conclusion

Our comparative study with seven low dose OC's, all containing about the same amount of ethinyl estradiol, but different types and doses of progestagens indicates that:

— Diane-35® does not adversely effect the metabolism parameters studied; the effect on HDL 2 and Apo A-1 seems to be *beneficial.*

— The increase of SHBG and CBG causes a decrease of the free, biologically active fraction of testosterone. This action is additive to the anti-androgenic action of cyproterone acetate on the androgen-receptor, and thus beneficial in the treatment of androgen-related phenomenon such as acne vulgaris and hypertrichosis.

References

[1] Anderson, D. X.: Sex hormone binding globulin. Clin. Endocrinol. **3** (1974) 69—96.

[2] Aydinlik, S., U. Lachnit-Fixson, J. Lehnert: Östrogenreduzierten Ovulationshemmer zur Akne Therapie. Fortschr. med. **104** (1986) 547—551.

[3] Byrne, G. C., Y. S. Perry, J. S. D. Winter: Steroid inhibitory effects upon human adrenal 3β-hydroxysteroid dehydrogenase activity. Clin. Endocrin. e Metabl. **62** (1986) 413.

[4] Elstein, M., Forword: J. of Obstet. e Gynaec. **4** (1984) (suppl. 2) S 73.

[5] Fanta, D.: Oral contraceptives in dermatology. In: Haspels, A. A., C. R. Kay, (eds.): International Symposium on Hormonal Contraception, pp. 50—56. Excerpta Medica, Amsterdam—Oxford 1978.

[6] Gordon, T., W. P. Castelli, M. C. Hjortland et al.: High density lipoprotein as a protective against coronary heart disease. Am. J. Med. **62** (1977) 707—714.

[7] Hammerstein, J., B. Cupceancu: Behandlung der Hirsutismus mit Cyproteronacetat. Dtsch. med. Wschr. **94** (1969) 829.

[8] Miller, N. E., O. H. Forde, D. S. Thelle et al.: The Tromso Heart Study. High density lipoprotein and coronary heart disease: a prospective casecontrol study. Lancet **1** (1977) 956—958.

[9] Tikkanen, M. J., E. A. Nikkila, T. Kuusi: Reduction of plasma high-density lipoprotein 2—cholesterol and increase of post heparin plasma hepatic lipase activity during progestin treatment. Clin. Chim. Acta. **115** (1981) 63—71.

[10] Van der Vange, N., H. J. Kloosterboer, A. A. Haspels: Effects of seven low dose combined oral Contraceptives on HDL subfraction. Brit. Journ. of Obst. e Gynaec. In press.

Antiandrogen therapy for signs of androgenization: an overview

A. E. Schindler

Among various compounds which exert antiandrogenic effects two main chemical groups can be discerned as shown in table 1.

Antiandrogens are compounds which interfere with the action of androgens in the target cell (competitive action at the androgen receptor). However none of the pure antiandrogens have proven very effective [10]. Therefore, antiandrogens with additional effects are of clinical interest and have found practical application. These effects are mediated by:

1. Hypothalamic-pituitary suppression (antigonadotropic, anticorticotropic) which leads to a decrease of ovarian and adrenal androgen secretion.
2. Changes in androgen metabolism produced by 5-alpha-reductase activity.

Compounds with progestational activity are of particular interest since they can achieve good menstrual cycle control when combined with estrogens. The latter can decrease androgen action by elevating the circulating steroid binding proteins and thereby reducing the levels of the circulating free androgens.

The nonsteroidal compounds flutamide and cimetidine have not gained clinical importance so far [17, 24]. However the steroids listed in table 1, have found varyingly wide clinical application. Cyproterone acetate is particularly widely used.

Up to now, a variety of regimens have been developed in an attempt to fulfill clinical requirements. Three of the steroids listed in table 1 will be considered more closely:

Table 1 Compounds with antiandrogenic effects

COMPOUND	CEMICAL STRUCTURE
Cimetidine	Nonsteroid
Flutamide	Nonsteroid
Chlormadinone acetate	Steroid/Gestagen
Cyproterone acetate	Steroid/Gestagen
Medrogestone	Steroid/Gestagen
Medroxyprogesterone acetate	Steroid/Gestagen
Megestrol acetate	Steroid/Gestagen
Spironolactone	Steroid/Aldosterone antagonist

1. Cyproterone acetate
2. Chlormadinone acetate
3. Spironolactone

The gestagens cyproterone acetate and chlormadinone acetate can be used in two ways:

1. Monotherapy
2. Combination therapy

Further more, monotherapy with gestagens alone can be carried out cyclicly or continuously.

1. Monotherapy

a. Cyclic antiandrogen therapy

Chlormadinone acetate in doses of 2 to 4 mg are given from days 15 to 24/26 of the cycle [13]. A similar regimen with cyproterone acetate to my knowledge has not been tested so far, but it appears possible to use 10 mg of cyproterone acetate from day 15 to 24 of the cycle.

The clinical antiandrogenic effect of this type of treatment is probably not substantial, but can be satisfactory in some individuals.

b. Continuous antiandrogen therapy

In postmenopausal women or after hysterectomy a daily doses of 10 to 100 mg cyproterone acetate seems to be effective. For the postmenopausal women such a treatment regimen avoids withdrawal bleeding encountered with estrogen/gestagen combinations. It also has a beneficial effect on androgenic symptomatology, alleviates climacteric symptoms, causes regression of abnormal proliferative states of the endometrium and the breast and protects against exaggerated bone loss [25].

2. Combinationtherapy

A variety of combinations of estrogens mainly with cyproterone acetate have been developed to treat signs of androgenization in women.

Monophasic preparations

Diane®
(21 tbls 0,05 mg ethinyl estradiol / 2 mg cyproterone acetate)

Diane-35®
(21 tbls 0,035 mg ethinyl estradiol / 2 mg cyproterone acetate)

Gestamestrol®
(21 tbls 0,1 mg Mestranol / 3 mg chlormadinone acetate)

Large clinical experiences with Diane® and Diane-35® has been gained [1, 13, 14, 16, 19, 20].

Biphasic preparations

Eunomin®
(11 tbls 0,1 mg mestranol, 10 tbls 0,1 mg mestranol / 2 mg chlomadinone acetate)

Neo-Eunomin®
(11 tbls 0,05 mg ethinyl estradiol / 1 mg chlormadinone acetate, 11 tbls 0,05 mg EE / 2 mg chlormadinone acetate)

Reverse sequential therapy

Because cyproterone acetate is accumulated when higher doses are used, a regimen was proposed which limits cyproterone acetate administration to days 5 to 14 of the cycle whereas ethinyl estradiol is given for 21 days. This was first published in 1969 [9]:

0,05 mg ethinyl estradiol days 5 to 24 of the cycle/
100.0 mg cyproterone acetate days 5 to 14 of the cycle

For own studies and treatment the following regimen was used [26]:

0,04 mg ethinyl estradiol (2 tbls Progynon C®), days 5 to 24 of the cycle,
100.0 mg cyproterone acetate (2 tbls Androcur®) days 5 to 14 of the cycle

In order to improve effectiveness, the daily dose can be increased up to 200 mg cyproterone acetate.

Several modifications of the principle of reverse sequential therapy have been proposed [18, 20]. Use of 4 mg estradiol valerate on days 5 to 24 or intramuscular injection of 10 mg estradiol valerate on days 5 and 14 of the cycle in combination with 100 mg cyproterone acetate on days 5 to 14 has been suggested.

Also the use of Diane® in combination with either 100 mg cyproterone acetate from days 5 to 14 of the cycle or with 10 mg cyproterone acetate for the first 15 days of Diane® treatment has been recommended [19, 21].

A further possibility of combined therapy is the use of 300 mg Depot-cyproterone acetate on day 5 with 40 to 50 μg ethinyl estradiol daily from day 5 to 24 of the cycle [18].

In cases with side effects of oral estrogen intake, a combination of percutaneous estradiol and oral cyproterone acetate has proven clinically effective. The regimen consists of 50 mg cyproterone acetate from day 5 to 25 of the cycle and 3 mg estradiol percutaneously from day 16 to 25 of the cycle. An exceptionally good clinical tolerance of this combination has been reported [15, 23].

Spironolactone

Spironolactone has been used intermittently for 3 weeks or continuously in doses of 50 to 200 mg. Since, however, cycle disturbances can be encountered it has been recommended that this substance be used together with estrogen/gestagen combinations in order to regulate the bleeding pattern as well as to improve effectiveness, and to provide a contraceptive effect [2, 3, 5, 7, 8, 16, 22, 27].

Because of reports of side effects the use of spironolactone in women with signs of androgenization will probably be prohibited in the future.

Hormonal contraceptives

In general, all hormonal contraceptive preparations can improve signs of androgenization in women. Because they are antigonadotropic and anticorticotropic they lead to a decrease of the circulating androgen levels. They can also cause an increase in steroid binding proteins and, therefore, reduction of the biologically active free androgen fraction. The extent of such an effect is dependent on the type and dose of the estrogen and gestagen used.

Preparations which use 19-nortestosterone derivatives as the gestagen will be less effective than other contraceptives depending upon the androgenic properties of the derivative and the dose of estrogen used [4, 6, 11, 12].

Conclusion

In the search for improved antiandrogen therapy emphasis should be directed not only towards the compounds themselves but also towards optimalization of estrogen/antiandrogen combinations. These should have a minimum of possible side effects (metabolic, hemostasiologic, cardiovascular) and a maximum of clinical effect on signs of androgenization in women. The development of Diane® and Diane-35® presents the result of such an approach.

References

[1] Aydinlik, S., U. Lachnit-Fixson, J. Lehnert: Östrogen-reduzierter Ovulationshemmer zur Aknetherapie. Fortschritte d. Medizin **104** (1986) 547—551.
[2] Boiselle, A., R. R. Tremblay: New therapeutic approach to the hirsute patient. Fert. Steril. **32** (1979) 276—279.
[3] Chapman, M. G., M. Dowsett, C. J. Dewhurst et al.: Spironolactone in combination with an oral contraceptive: an alternative treatment for hirsutism. Brit. J. Obstet. Gynec **92** (1985) 983—985.
[4] Cullberg, G., L. Hamberger, L. A. Mattson et al.: Positiver Effect oraler Kontrazep-

tion bei Hirsutismus und PCO-Syndrom. Acta Obstet. Gynecol. Scand **64** (1985) 195—202.

[5] Cumming, D. C., J. C. Yang, R. V. Rebar et al.: Treatment of hirsutism with spironolactone. JAMA **247** (1982) 1295—1298.

[6] Dewis, P., P. Petsos, M. Newman et al.: The treatment of hirsutism with combination of desogestrel and ethinyl estradiol. Clin. Endocrinol. **22** (1985) 29—36.

[7] Dorrington-Ward, P., A. C. E. McCartney, S. Holland et al.: The effect of spironolactone on hirsutism and female androgen metabolism. Clin. Endocrinol. **23** (1985) 161—167.

[8] Givens, R. J.: Treatment of hirsutism with spironolactone. Fert. Steril **43** (1985) 841—843.

[9] Hammerstein, J., B. Cupceancu: Behandlung des Hirsutismus mit Cyproteronazetat. Dtsch. Med. Wschr. **94** (1969) 829—834.

[10] Hammerstein, J., S. Nigam, M. Droste-Velm et al.: Experience with antiandrogens in the treatment of hirsutism. In: Bruchowsky, N., A. Chapdelaine, F. Neumann (eds.): Regulation of androgen action, pp. 115—117, Brückner, Berlin 1985.

[11] Hancock, K. W., M. J. Leval: The use of estrogen, progestogen preparations in the treatment of hirsutism in the female. J. Obstet. Gynaec. Brit. Cwlth **81** (1974) 804—811.

[12] Hoffmann, E., H. G. Meiers, A. Hubbes: Wirkungen von Antikonzeptiva auf Alopecia androgenetica, Seborrhoea oleosa, Akne vulgaris und Hirsutismus. Dtsch. Med. Wschr. **99** (1974) 2121—2157.

[13] Kaiser, E.: Behandlung von Androgenisierungserscheinungen der Frau (hormonell). Ärztl. Kosmetologie **15** (1985) 260—271.

[14] Kaiser, E.: Klinische Erfahrungen mit Diane-35®, der zur Zeit niedrigst dosierte antiandrogenwirkende hormonale Ovulationshemmer bei leichten bis mittelstarken Androgenisierungserscheinungen der Frau. Geburtsh. Frauenheilkunde **46** (1986) 738—742.

[15] Kuttenn, F., C. Rigaud, F. Wright et al.: Treatment of hirsutism by oral cyproterone acetate and percutaneous estradiol. J. Clin. Endocrinol. Metab. **51** (1980) 1107—1111.

[16] Lobo, R. A., D. Shoupe, P. Scrafini et al.: The effect of two doses of spironolactone on serum androgens and anagen hair inhirsutism. Fert. Steril. **43** (1985) 200—205.

[17] Molinatti, G. M., M. Messina, C. Manieri et al.: Current approached to the treatment of virilizing syndromes. In: Molinatti, G. M., L. Martini, V. H. T. James (eds.): Androgenization in women, pp. 179—193, Raven Press, New York 1983.

[18] Moltz, L., F. Haase, U. Schwartz et al.: Die Behandlung androgenisierter Frauen mit intramuskulär applizierbarem Cyproteronazetat. Geburtsh. Frauenheilk. **43** (1983) 281—287.

[19] Moltz, L., E. Kaiser: Mittelhochdosierte orale Cyproteronazetat-Therapie bei Frauen mit mittelgradig ausgeprägten Androgenisierungserscheinungen. Geburtsh. Frauenheilk. **44** (1984) 47—52.

[20] Moltz, L., U. Schwartz, J. Hammerstein: Die klinische Anwendung von Antiandrogenen bei der Frau. Der Gynäkologe **13** (1980) 1—17.

[21] Neumann, F., S. Aydinlik, U. Lachnit-Fixon: The treatment of androgen-induced or mediated disorders of the skin with cyproterone acetate. In: Bruchowsky, N., A. Chapdelaine, F. Neumann (eds.): Regulation of androgen action, pp. 109—113, Brückner, Berlin 1985.

[22] Pittaway, D. E., W. S. Maxsid, A. C. Wentz: Spironolactone in combination drug therapy for unresponsive hirsutism. Fert. Steril. **43** (1985) 878—882.

[23] Rigaud, C., M. Vincens, J. Mowszowicz et al.: Mecanisme d'action de l'acetate de

cyproterone dans le traitement de l'hirsutisme. Ann. d'Endoconologie **44** (1983) 387—392.

[24] Schindler, A. E.: Antiandrogene in der Gynäkologie. Sexualmedizin **5** (1977) 360—366.

[25] Schindler, A. E.: Prävention in Gynäkologie und Geburtshilfe. Terramed communications, Überlingen 1986.

[26] Schindler, A. E., K. Mangold, E. Friederich et al.: Therapy of androgenetic symptomatology with cyproterone acetate and ethinyl estradiol. Arch. Gynäk. **225** (1978) 103—107.

[27] Shapiro, G., S. Evron: A novel use of spironolactone: treatment of hirsutism. J. Clin. Endocrinol. Metab. **51** (1980) 429—432.

I Pharmacology and physiology

Pharmacological aspects of cyproterone acetate

F. Neumann

Introduction

The pharmacology of cyproterone acetate has been reviewed in many articles [6, 5, 16, 4, 15, 10]. In this short paper I will summarize the most important pharmacological aspects and I will discuss those activity patterns, which are important for the treatment of androgen-induced or mediated disorders of the female skin in detail.

For the indication under discussion the activity pattern of cyproterone acetate is of great importance. Cyproterone acetate has

1. antiandrogenic
2. progestagenic and
3. antigonadotrophic

properties. This antiandrogen has no androgenic or estrogenic properties at all as has been postulated.

Chemistry

Chemically, cyproterone acetate is a hydroxyprogesterone derivative. Of major importance for the antiandrogenic action is the methylene substituent of the steroid molecule (fig. 1).

Although quite a number of derivatives display antiandrogenic activity, none match the potency of cyproterone acetate (fig. 1). Even at present, cyproterone acetate is the most potent antiandrogen known in intact individuals.

Since the free alcohols of hydroxyprogesterone derivatives are devoid of progestational properties, it was surprising that cyproterone (the free alcohol of cyproterone acetate) still displayed antiandrogenic activity, although this activity was less potent than that of cyproterone acetate. This is also true for all other free alcohols of antiandrogenic derivatives of cyproterone acetate [19].

Cyproterone acetate	
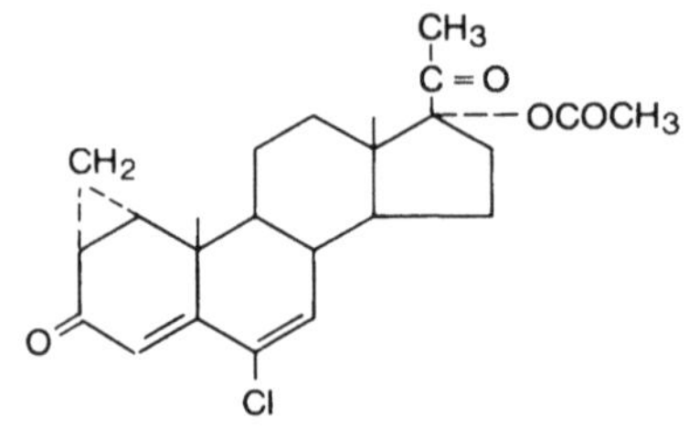	
Structural changes of Cyproterone acetate	Relativ potency compared with Cyproterone acetate
- 4-H + 4-Cl	1
- 1α,2α-CH_2 + 1-H + 2-H	0,3
- 1α,2α-CH_2 + 1α-CH_3 + 2-H	0,3
- 3-O + 3-OH + 3-H	0,9
- 6-Cl + 6-H	0,6
- 17-OAc + 17-OH	0,5
D-homo 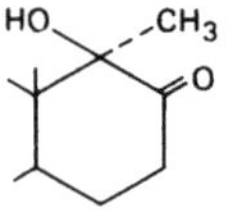	0,7

Fig. 1 Chemical structure of cyproterone acetate and antiandrogenic potency of some cyproterone acetate derivatives.

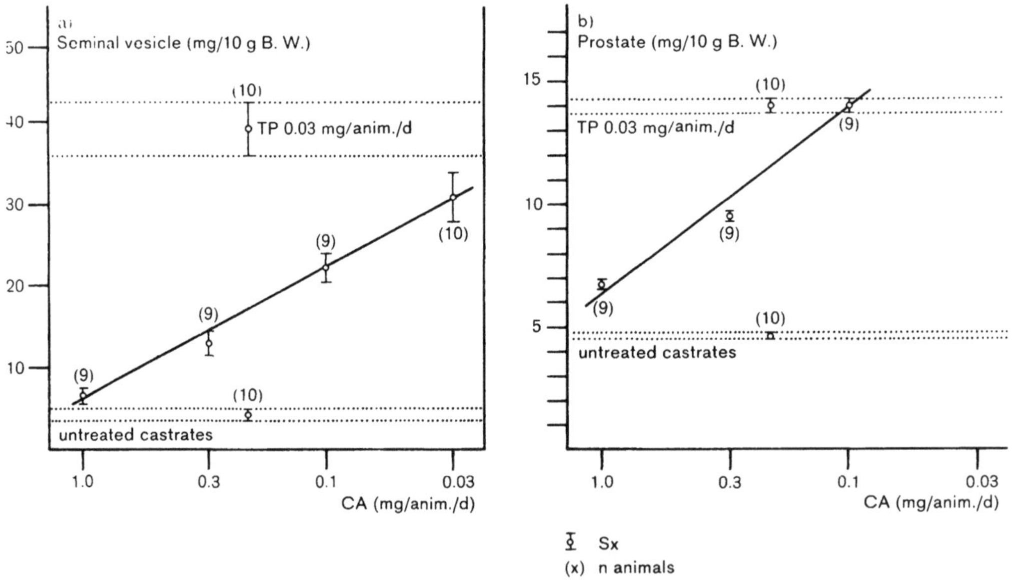

Fig. 2 Inhibition of the stimulating effect of 0.03 mg testosterone propionate on the seminal vesicle (a) and prostate weight (b) in castrated mice by administration of cyproterone acetate in increasing dosages.

Mechanism of action

Cyproterone acetate was recognised as an antiandrogen because it feminized male fetuses [11, 7]. From the beginning it was considered most likely that feminization was induced by inhibiting the effect of androgens at the target organ level. That this was, indeed, the case is illustrated in figure 2, which shows the results of a very historic experiment.

In this experiment, mice were castrated and given replacement therapy, the exogenous administration of an androgen. When cyproterone acetate was administered concurrently, the effect of the exogenous androgen, e. g., increase of the weight of the prostate and seminal vesicles, was inhibited in a dose-dependent manner.

This finding suggested the presence of a competitive antagonism, i. e., an antiandrogenic effect.

The molecular mechanism of action of cyproterone acetate and of antiandrogens is summarized in figures 3 and 4.

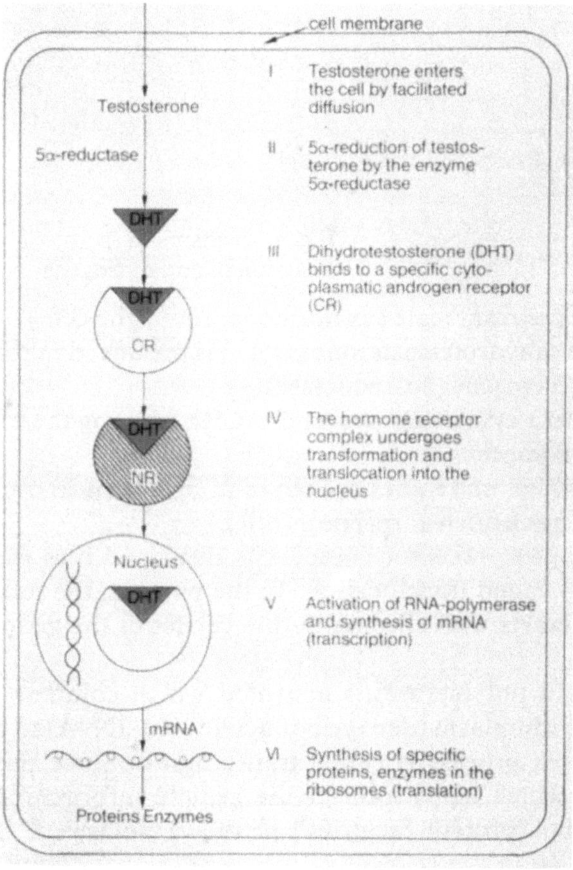

Fig. 3 Mechanism of action of androgens

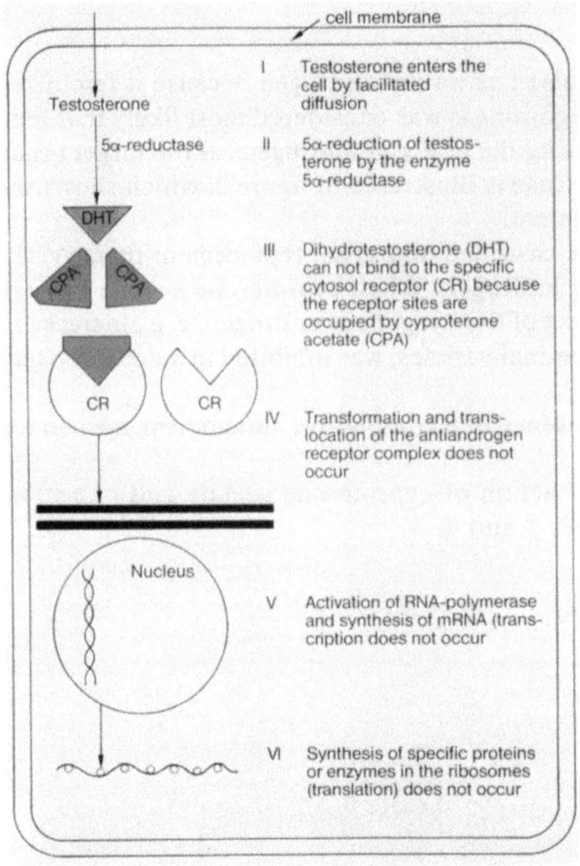

Fig. 4 Mechanism of action of antiandrogens

I. Testosterone (T), the most important male sex hormone, enters the cell.

II. The testosterone metabolite dihydrotestosterone (DHT) is produced in the cell under the influence of an enzyme (5α-reductase).

III. Dihydrotestosterone binds to a cytoplasmic receptor (CR), creating the dihydrotestosterone receptor complex.

IV. The hormone receptor complex undergoes a change in its chemical and physical properties. It becomes a nuclear receptor (NR).
The dihydrotestosterone nuclear receptor complex is displaced into the cell nucleus. This process is called translocation. In the nucleus, the hormone receptor complex interacts with chromatin (the carrier of the genotype).

V. An enzyme (ribonucleic acid polymerase) is activated which communicates the information of the idioplasm (deoxyribonucleic acid, DNA) to a ribonucleic acid (RNA). This process is called transcription. Since this RNA acts as a messenger which helps transfer the genetic information from the cell nucleus to the "protein factories" in the cytoplasm, it is known as messenger RNA.

VI. The information carried by the messenger RNA is translated at the "protein factories", the ribosomes. This process is called translation.

Thus, the actual hormone effect is achieved by the synthesis of certain protein substances.

Antiandrogens compete with dihydrotestosterone for the cytoplasmic receptor. The antiandrogen receptor complex is not translocated into the cell nucleus.

Antiandrogenic properties

With few exceptions, such as effects on libido of commonly used laboratory animals, cyproterone acetate inhibits the action of endogenous and exogenous androgens on all androgen target organ systems these include the prostate, seminal vesicles, testes, and the vas deferens. This antiandrogen also antagonises less sex-specific effects of androgens such as, for example, ossification of the epiphyseal cartilage, sebaceous gland function and skin thickness (for review see [10]). Table 1 summarizes these effects.

Table 1 Effects of cyproterone acetate

Organ system/function	Effect of cyproterone acetate
Accessory sex glands	Atrophy, loss of secretory activity
Spermatogenesis	Inhibition
Libido and potency	Loss of libido (except in some rodents)
Puberty	Inhibition of onset of puberty
Male sexual differentiation	Feminization
Longitudinal bone growth	Retardation
Bone maturation, ossification	Retardation
Sebaceous gland function	Inhibition

I would like to discuss a few examples. The effects of CPA on the normal prostate correspond to those of surgical castration. Proliferative and secretory activity cease completely. Characteristic enzymes (e. g., acid phosphatase) and constituents of the prostate (e. g., zinc) are no longer determinable [8, 14]. An example of this is given in figure 5 which shows the complete atrophy of a dog prostate after combined treatment with an androgen and cyproterone acetate. The effect corresponds to that of surgical castration.

Since spermatogenesis is also an androgen-dependent process, cyproterone acetate also interfers with this process [9]. An example is given in figure 6, which shows the histology of dog testes.

A consistent finding is that under medium doses only spermatid maturation (spermiogenesis) is initially affected. Under higher doses meiosis fails to take place; secondary spermatocytes are then the most advanced stages of spermatogenesis. Under extremely high doses, the tubules are completely depopulated and, apart from Sertoli cells, only spermatogonia and early spermatocyte forms are recognizable.

And as a last example we have the effect of CPA on another more sex-specific organ or function: the effect on onset of puberty and libido [17].

The onset of puberty can be delayed in both animals and humans. Precocious puberty is therefore, an indication for cyproterone acetate [for review see 1, 6]. One relevant animal experiment is shown in figure 7.

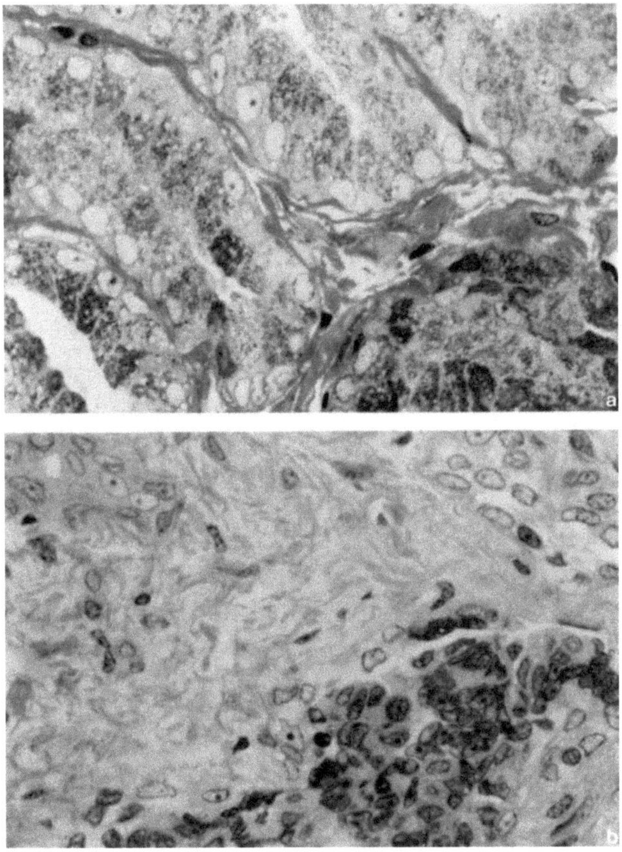

Fig. 5A Prostate of castrated dogs (semi-thin sections) after 6 months' treatment with 25 mg 3 α, 17β-androstanediol weekly. The prostate displays marked scretory activity.

Fig. 5B Additional treatment with 600 mg cyproterone acetate weekly. The secretory activity has ceased completely, the prostate is atrophic — comparable with the effect of castration.
Staining: Laczko
Magnification: 1600x

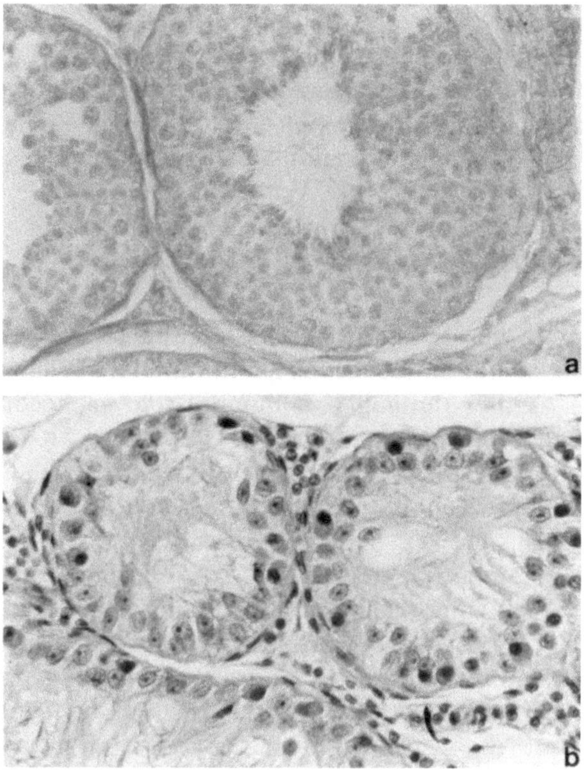

Fig. 6A Dog testes. Control.

Fig. 6B After approx. 12 months' oral administration of 100 mg/day/kg body weight cyproterone acetate. Note the tubular atrophy and depopulation of the germinal epithelium;
meiosis is inhibited.
Staining: Haematoxilin-eosin
Magnification: 265x

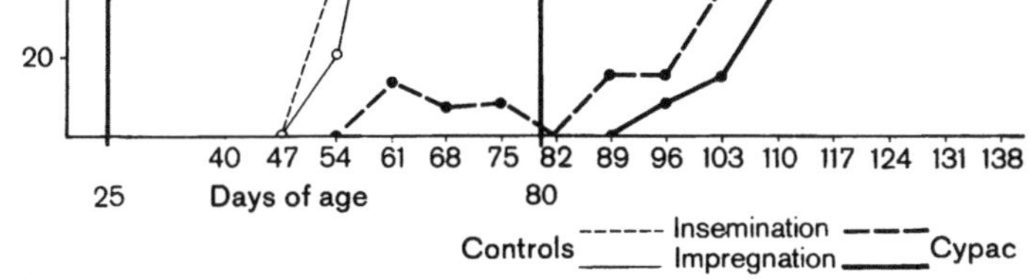

Fig. 7 Influence of peripubertal cyproterone acetate (CPA) treatment on the reproductive performance of male rats.

The onset of puberty in rats is delayed by treatment with cyproterone acetate. At the same time, the stimulating effect of androgens on ossification of the epiphyseal cartilage is inhibited so that the phase of growth of the long bones is prolonged. Libido is also inhibited in some, but not all animal species and in men. Hypersexuality is then another indication for cyproterone acetate [3].

Effect on sebaceous gland function

In regards to the disorders of the skin under discussion, the most important effect of cyproterone acetate is that on sebaceous gland function. It has been demonstrated in numerous studies (animal and human) that sebaceous gland function is androgen dependent. It is also known that increased sebaceous gland function is of causal significance for the development of acne and seborrhoea. A relationship exists between the rate of sebum secretion and the severity of acne [for review see 2].

I would like to quickly demonstrate the effect of cyproterone acetate on sebaceous gland function by showing data from two animal experiments.

Table 2 summarizes the effect of cyproterone acetate on sebaceous gland function in mice. The cell volume of castrated, androgen-replaced animals was four times that of intact, untreated controls. Treatment with 1 mg cyproterone acetate every second day for four weeks led to an 80% reduction in the volume of sebaceous gland tissue. The stimulatory effect of testosterone propionate is inhibited by the simultaneous administration of cyproterone acetate.

A second example is shown in figure 8. In this case, the hamster ear model

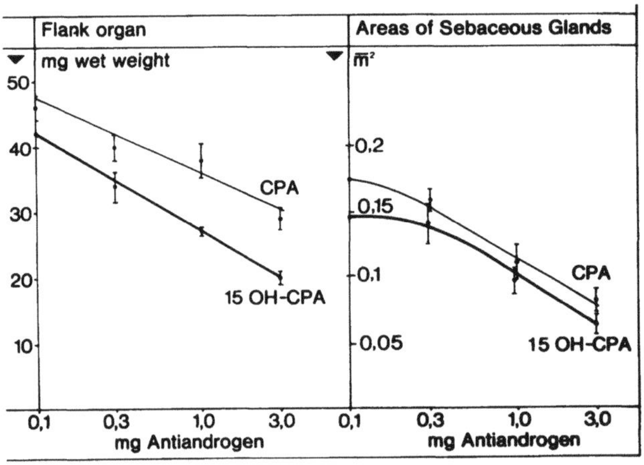

Fig. 8 Effect of three weeks systemic administration of cyproterone acetate (CPA) and its main metabolite, 15-OH-cyproterone acetate (15-OH-CPA) on the weight of the flank organ and on the sebaceous gland areas in the ear of castrated male hamsters treated with 0.1 mg testosterone proponate/day/animal.

Table 2 Evaluation of effts of CPA on sebaceous glands in mice (dorsal skin sections)

Group	Number of animals	Number of alveoli per cm skin section	Number of cells per alveolus	Diameter of cells (μm)	Volume of cells (μm^3)	Total volume of sebaceous gland tissue μm^3/cm skin section X 10^{-3}	in % of controls
1. Intact male treated with vehicle only	8	19 ± 8	6.9 ± 0.98	15.3 ± 0.4	1866 ± 113	262 ± 153	100
2. Intact male treated* with 1 mg CA** per animal	7	9 ± 5.8	5.0 ± 0.6	11.5 ± 1.9	862 ± 431	49 ± 45	18.8
3. Castrated male, treated* with 0.5 mg TP*** per animal	8	57 ± 17.4	8.8 ± 1.2	15.8 ± 0.35	2065 ± 140	1030 ± 307	391
4. Castrated male, treated* with 0.5 mg TP*** and 1 mg CA** per animal	6	25 ± 6.9	5.5 ± 0.83	13.8 ± 0.8	1390 ± 227	196 ± 71	75

*) Substance solution injected i.m. every other day for 4 weeks
**) CA = cyproterone acetate
***) TP = testosterone propionate

was used to demonstrate the effect of cyproterone acetate and its main metabolite, 15-hydroxycyproterone acetate, on sebaceous gland function. The areas of sebaceous glands were measured by means of planimetry. The weight of the flank organ (a large gland with holocrine secretion) was also determined. It is interesting that the main metabolite, 15-hydroxycyproterone acetate, is more potent than the parent compound.

Progestational properties

The progestational potency of cyproterone acetate is important for its clinical use, especially in women.

Cyproterone acetate has been shown in classical tests to be a potent progestin. It is one of the most effective progestins in the group of hydroxyprogesterone derivatives (Wiechert, Neumann 1965) and has about the same range of effects as progesterone. Table 3 lists some of its typical progestational effects.

Figure 9 presents, for various progestins, a comparison of the oral threshold values in the Clauberg test in the rabbit with the oral transformation doses in the Kaufmann test in woman. Although some of the data for the Kaufmann test are highly inaccurate, it can still be seen that a highly significant correlation exists between the efficacies observed in the two test models. The clinical efficacy of cyproterone acetate is exceeded only by that of D-norgestrel (levonorgestrel) and norgestrel. It should be mentioned that cyproterone acetate displays a depot effect in the Clauberg test: 13 days after subcutaneous administration of 5 mg, an effect can still be demonstrated at the level of the endomet-

Table 3 Progestational effects of cyproterone acetate

Test	Effect
Clauberg test (rabbit)	Endometrial transformation
Clauberg test (dog)	Endometrial transformation
Maintenance of pregnancy in castrated rats	Pregnancy maintenance in combination with estrogens
Delay of implantation (rat)	Implantation delayed (delayed nidation)
Oxytocin-induced abortion (rabbit)	Counteraction of the oxytocin-induced abortion
Parturition	Inhibition of parturition
Antiestrogenic effect in the periphery (e.g., sialic acid test in the mouse uterus)	Counteraction of estrogen effects in the vagina and uterus
Fertilization inhibition test in the rabbit (test for influence on cervical factor)	Inhibition of fertilization on artificial vaginal insemination
Experimentally induced permanent estrus in rats	Interruption of the permanent estrus

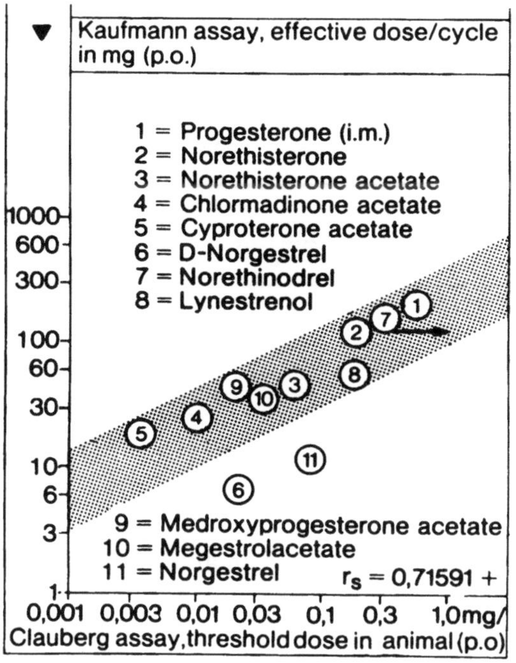

Fig. 9 Progestational potencies. Comparison of the oral transformation dose (Kaufmann test) in women with the oral threshold value (Clauberg test) in rabbits.

rium. This weak depot effect is also of clinical significance, particularly for the high-dose therapy of hirsutism.

Antiestrogenic properties

In pharmacological tests, at least, the antiestrogenic effect of cyproterone acetate correlates with its peripheral progestational activity. Like other progestins, cyproterone acetate is able to suppress experimentally induced permanent estrus in rats.

In castrated mice, estrogens administration leads to a reduction of vaginal content of sialic acid in the vagina. The changes are comparable to those in the cervical secretion of women under estrogen domination. The administration of progestins leads to mucification of the vaginal epithelium and an increase of the sialic acid content as an expression of an increased mucin content.

Table 4 shows the effective dose range for some progestins. From this table it can also be seen that efficacy in this model correlates well with that at the "mini-pill" dose in women. Cyproterone acetate is also quite potent in this assay.

Table 4 Comparison of the antiestrogenic efficacy of various progestins in the subcutaneous sialic acid test in the mouse with the oral 'mini-pill' dose in the woman

Progestin	Sialic acid test in the mouse		'Mini-pill' dose in the woman	
	Dose range (mg/day)	Relative efficacy (Covariance analysis: Chlormadinone acetate = 1)	Dose range (mg/day)	Relative efficacy (Covariance analysis: Chlormadinone acetate = 1)
Norethisterone acetate	10 – 100	8	0.6	1.7
Levonorgestrel	0.3– 10	83	0.03	33
Chlormadinone acetate	30 –1000	1	=1	1
Cyproterone acetate	30 – 300	1	<1	> 1

Antigonadotrophic potency

Like all other progestins, cyproterone acetate has an antigonadotrophic effect. This effect is most apparent in females, but also occurs in males at higher doses. Inhibition of ovulation is, for example, an expression of antigonadotrophic activity.

The antiovulatory effectiveness of various progestins in women and in rats is shown in figure 10.

The oral effective dose 100 of cyproterone acetate is about 1 mg/day in women.

Glucocorticoid-like properties

Cyproterone acetate and some chemically related steroids have glucocorticoid-like properties in animals [for review see 10].

For example, the weights of the adrenals and thymus decrease in rats and other species of laboratory animals. The adrenal atrophy is due to reduced secretion of adrenocorticotropic hormone (ACTH) and results in the reduced synthesis and secretion of glucocorticoids. For example, corticosterone levels fall in the rat and hydrocortisone in the guinea-pig. On the other hand, CPA has no antiinflammatory properties (granuloma pouch test) and is also ineffective in the eosinophil test. Thus cyproterone acetate and similar antiandrogens display only some of the typical effects of glucocorticoids. No sign of secondary adrenal insufficiency has been seen in any study.

On clinical use, glucocorticoid effects apparently become manifest only during high-dose (more than 80—100 mg/m^2 body area) CPA therapy of children with precocious puberty. These children fail to display signs of secondary adrenal insufficiency [for review see 1, 6].

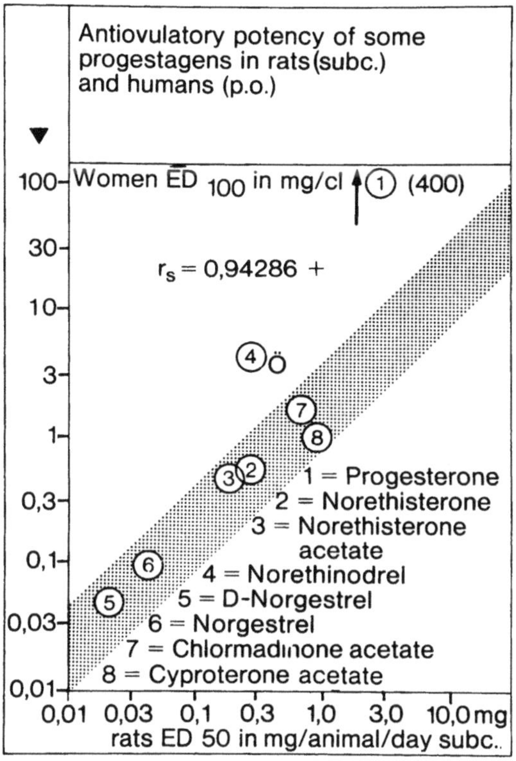

Fig. 10 Antiovulatory efficacy of various progestins. Comparison of the oral ovulation-inhibiting dose in women with subcutaneous doses in rats.

Fetal Feminization

1. What kind of intersexuality is induced by cyproterone acetate?
The specific form of intersexuality induced by antiandrogens occurs spontaneously in humans and also in some other species and is called testicular feminization.

Figure 11 shows such a person; these individuals are genetically and gonadally male, but they lack an internal efferent genital tract. The vagina ends blindly. In general, the presence of intersexuality is recognised in these persons only when menstruation fails to occur during puberty (absence of a uterus).

Figure 12 shows schematically the form of intersexuality which results in the male sex when androgens do not become effective in the phase of sexual differentiation. The reconstruction is based on serial sections of dog foetuses from the 45th day of foetal development. The testes have not yet descended at this time. It can be seen that the foetus whose mother was treated with cyproterone acetate (10 mg/kg) from the 25th to the 44th day displays normal testes. However, there is no internal efferent genital tract, either male or female, i. e. no com-

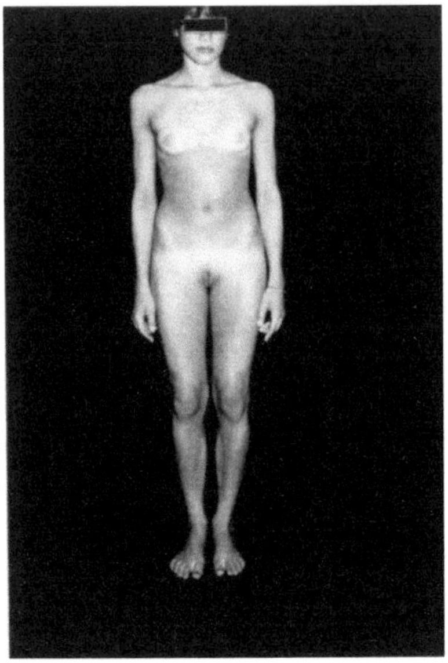

Fig. 11 Syndrome of testicular feminisation (reproduced with kind permission of Prof. Breckwoldt, Gynaecological Clinic of the University of Freiburg). The individuals are genetically and gonadally male, but they consistently lack an efferent genital tract. The vagina ends blindly. In general, intersexuality in these individuals is recognised only at puberty, when menstruation fails to occur (absence of a uterus).

munication exists from the testes to the body surface. Accessory sex glands such as prostate and seminal vesicles are absent and, instead, there is a blind-end vagina. The external genitalia are female. Figure 13 shows the external genitalia of an adult feminized dog (note the well-developed vagina) [for review see 12, 13, 11].

2. What is the therapeutic range regarding the risk of feminization of a human fetus when the mother is taking a cyproterone acetate-containing preparation during the critical phase of differentiation?

This question is asked very often. First of all, patients do not become pregnant when taking the preparation containing 2 mg cyproterone acetate and 50 or 35 μg ethinyl estradiol (Diane®).

However, it happens that a woman starts taking this drug after she is already pregnant.

There is, of course, no exact answer to this question and we must rely on the results of animal experiments. We have, however, tried to calculate the therapeutic range for the progestational components of several oral contraceptives in respect to the risk of feminisation of cyproterone acetate and the risk of virilisation of norethisterone acetate and levonorgestrel. The results are given in tables 5 and 6.

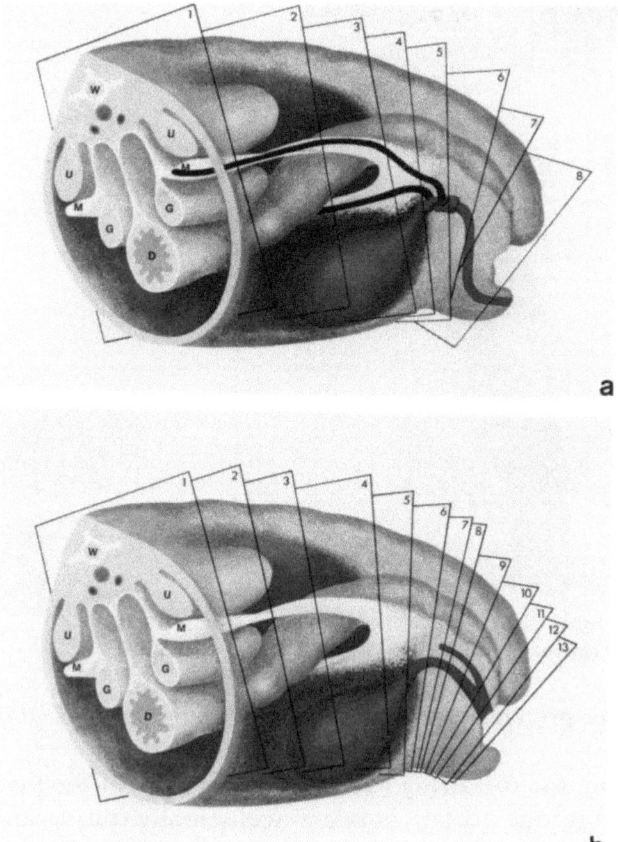

Fig. 12 Schematic presentation of the intersexuality which occurs in male foetuses whose mothers were treated with cyproterone acetate during the critical phase of sexual differentiation. This drawing is based on serial sections through dog foetuses (45th day)

a) Normal male control
b) Feminized male foetus (the mother had been treated with cyproterone acetate form day 23 to day 44 with 10 mg/kg/day i. m.).

Note the absence of the internal genital duct system, the absence of a prostate, and the presence of external female genitalia including the development of a blind-end vagina.

As is shown in table 5, the lowest dose which virilizes or feminizes rat fetuses is in the same range for all three compounds.

In table 6 the therapeutic range was obtained by deviding the calculated virilizing or fiminizing dose in animals (based on a mg/kg dose) by the progestogenic content (in mg of the tablet). This admittedly very schematic procedure produces a therapeutic latitude of 50 for the preparation with norethisterone

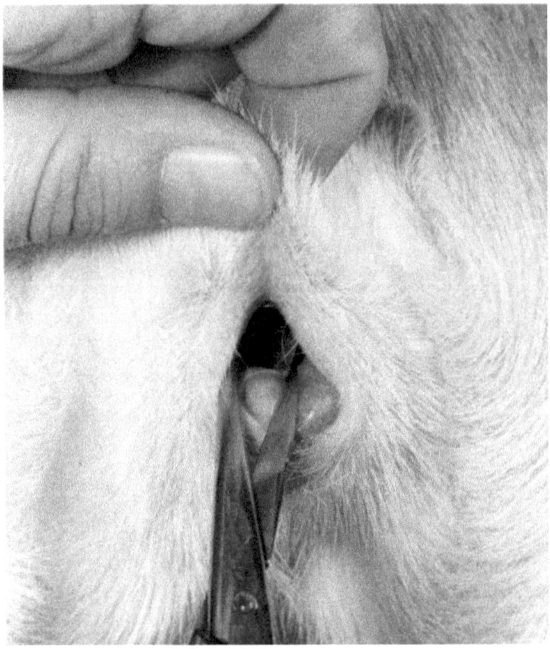

Fig. 13 Adult feminized male dog
(treatment of the mother as described in fig. 12).

acetate, of 240 for the preparation containing norgestrel and of 100 for Diane®.

With all due caution, the following can perhaps be said: If the preparation containing 2 mg cyproterone acetate is taken accidentally during an existing pregnancy, the risk of feminisation of a male fetus is probably not greater than the risk of virilisation of a female fetus when another oral contraceptive is

Table 5 Calculation of the risk of feminization or virilization of oral contraceptives based on the determination of the lowest dose which decreases or enlarges the anogenital distance in rat foetuses

Substance	Commercial preparation	Progestogen dose (mg/tablet)	Lowest dose which feminizes or virilizes rat foetuses (mg/animal s.c.)
Norethisterone acetate	Anovlar®	4.0	≈ 1.0
Norgestrel	Eugynon®	0.25	≈ 0.3
Cyproterone acetate	Diane®	2.0	≈ 1.0

Table 6 Calculation of the risk feminization or virilization of oral contraceptives in humans

Substance	Commercial preparation	Conversion of the rat foetusfeminising or virilising dose to man (mg/50 kg body weight)	'Therapeutic range' (referred to the progestogen dose/tablet)
Norethisterone acetate	Anovlar®	≈200	≈ 50
Norgestrel	Eugynon®	≈ 60	≈240
Cyproterone acetate	Diane®	≈200	≈100

taken under the same circumstances. We now know of 16 pregnancies (boys) where the mothers had taken Diane® during the whole critical phase of differentiation. All the boys born were normal and this seems to us much more conclusive than calculation of therapeutic range based on animal experiments.

The situation is probably different when the high-dose preparation (100 mg) is taken during pregnancy. Therapeutic range calculated was at a factor of only 2.

Conclusion and summary

Cyproterone acetate was the first antiandrogen to be introduced to clinical use. We have had almost 25 years of pharmacological experience with this antiandrogen.

Because increased sebaceous gland function is of causal significance for the development of acne and seborhoea, the strong inhibitory effect of cyproterone acetate on sebaceous glands gives the rational basis for these indications.

Cyproterone acetate is especially suitable for the treatment of these skin disorders because of its particular spectrum of activities: antiandrogenic, progestogenic, antigonadotropic.

References

[1] Girard, J., H. Helge, K. E. v. Mühlendahl: Treatment of idiopathic precocious puberty with cyproterone acetate. Proceedings of a Discussion, Berlin 1977. Horm. Res. (Basel) **9** (1978) 301—312.

[2] Hammerstein, J., U. Lachnit-Fixson, F. Neumann et al. (eds.): Androgenization in Women—Acne, Seborrhoe, Androgenetic Alopecia and Hirsutism. Excerpta Medica, Amsterdam, Oxford, Princeton 1980.

[3] Horn, H. J.: Administration of antiandrogens in hypersexuality and sexual deviations. In: Eichler, O., A. Farah, H. Herken et al. (eds.): Androgens II and Antiandrogens. Handbook of Experimental Pharmacology XXXV/2, chapt. VIII, pp. 543—562.

[4] Neumann, F.: Pharmacological basis for clinical use of antiandrogens. VI. International Congress on Hormonal Steroids, Jerusalem/Israel, September 5—10, 1982. J. Steroid Biochem. **19** (1983) 391—401.
[5] Neumann, F.: Experimental basis for the clinical use of antiandrogens. In: Bruchovsky, N., A. Chapdelaine, F. Neumann (eds.): Regulation of Androgen Action. Proceedings of an Intern. Symposium, Montreal 1984, pp. 43—50. Kongreßdruck R. Brückner, Berlin 1985.
[6] Neumann, F.: Pharmacology and clinical uses of cyproterone acetate. In: Furr, B. J. A., A. E. Wakeling (eds.): Pharmacology and Clinical Uses of Inhibitors of Hormone Secretion and Action, pp. 132—159. Baillière Tindall, London, Philadelphia, Toronto 1987.
[7] Neumann, F. H. Hamada: Intrauterine Feminisierung männlicher Rattenfeten durch das stark gestagen wirksame 6-chlor- 6.-1.2-methylen-17-hydroxyprogesteronacetat. 10. Symp. Dtsch. Ges. für Endokrinologie, Wien 1963, S. 301—304. Springer Verlag, Berlin 1964.
[8] Neumann, F., G. H. Jacobi: Antiandrogens in tumour therapy. Clin. Oncol. **1** (1982) 41—64.
[9] Neumann, F., B. Schenck: Antiandrogens: Basic concepts and clinical trials. In: Cunningham, G. R., W.-B. Schill, E. S. E. Hafez (eds.): Regulation of Male Fertility, pp. 93—104. Martinus Nijhoff Publishers bv, The Hague, Boston, London 1980.
[10] Neumann, F., H. Steinbeck: Antiandrogens. In: Eichler, O., A. Farah, H. Herken (eds.): Handbook of Experimental Pharmacology, pp. 235—484. Springer Verlag, Berlin, Heidelberg, New York 1974.
[11] Neumann, F., R. von Berswordt-Wallrabe, W. Elger: Aspects of androgen-dependant events as studied by antiandrogens. Rec. Progr. Horm. Res. **26** (1970) 337—410.
[12] Neumann, F., W. Elger, H. Steinbeck: Drug-induced intersexuality in mammals. Ann. Conference of the Society for the Study of Fertility, Newcastle 1968. J. Repro. Fert., Suppl. 7 (1969), 9—24.
[13] Neumann, F., W. Elger, H. Steinbeck: Antiandrogens and reproductive development. Phil. Trans. R. Soc. London, Series B, **259** (1970) 179—184.
[14] Neumann, F., K. D. Richter, B. Schenck et al.: Action of anti-androgens on accessory sexual glands. In: Schröder, F. H., H. J. de Voogt (eds.): Steroid Receptors, Metabolism and Prostatic Cancer, pp. 22—40.
Excerpta Medica, Amsterdam, Oxford, Princeton 1980.
[15] Neumann, F., A. Schleusener, M. Albring: Pharmacology of antiandrogens. In: Hammerstein, J., U. Lachnit-Fixson, F. Neumann (eds.): Androgenization in Women—Acne, Seborrhoe, Androgenetic Alopecia and Hirsutism, pp. 147—192. Excerpta Medica, Amsterdam, Oxford, Princeton 1980.
[16] Schleusener, A., M. Albring, F. Neumann: Pharmacology of old and new antiandrogens. In: Jeffcoate, S. L. (ed.): Androgens and Anti-androgen Therapy, Vol. 1, chapt. 4, pp. 71—93. John Wiley & Sons, Chechester, New York, Brisbane 1982.
[17] Steinbeck, H., F. Neumann: Effect of cyproterone acetate on puberty. J. Reprod. Fert. **26** (1971) 59—63.
[18] Wiechert, R., F. Neumann: Gestagene Wirksamkeit von 1-Methyl- und 1.2-Methylen-Steroiden.
IV. Mitteilung: 1-Methyl-Steroide 1.
Arzneimittelforsch. (Drug Res.) **15** (1965) 244—246.
[19] Wiechert, R., H. Steinbeck, W. Elger et al.: Wirkungen und Struktur neuer antiandrogener Steroide. Arzneimittelforsch. **17** (1967) 1103—1116.

Pharmacokinetics of cyproterone acetate and ethinyl estradiol in smoking and non-smoking women during treatment with Diane-35®

Chr. Zurth, U. Täuber

1. Introduction

Cyproterone acetate (CPA) is a potent antiandrogen with progestogenic activity [14, 15], which is used in men in the treatment of sexual deviations and prostate carcinoma, and in women in the treatment of androgenic symptoms and hirsutism [5, 12, 14].

For therapy of androgenic symptoms and hirsutism, three different therapeutic regimens have been established or were proposed [12, 13, 14]

(1) Low dose therapy with an oral contraceptive (OC) containing 2 mg CPA and 35 μg ethinylestradiol.

(2) Medium dose therapy by one intramuscular injection of 300 mg CPA per cycle.

(3) High oral dose therapy by 10 administrations of 100 mg CPA from day one to ten of the cycle together with Diane-35®.

The pharmacokinetics of CPA has been studied comprehensively in male volunteers and male patients as well as in female volunteers and female patients [3, 4, 6, 7, 9].

In the present investigation the time-course of the concentrations of CPA, of sex hormone binding globulin (SBHG) and of corticosteroid binding globulin (CBG) in the plasma was followed during one treatment cycle with Diane-35® in female volunteers. Additionally, the time-course of the active ingredients CPA and ethinylestradiol (EE_2) after the first and after the last administration was studied in greater detail.

Cigarette smoking is known to induce drug metabolising enzymes in the liver [2, 10, 19, 20, 21]. Since CPA and EE_2 are eliminated from the body by phase I biotransformation, the influence of cigarette smoking on the pharmacokinetics of CPA and EE_2 was investigated by comparing groups of non-smoking and smoking female volunteers.

2. Subjects and methods

2.1 Study design and volunteers

The trial was designed as a group comparison between eight non-smoking (age 29.4 ± 4.3 yr, weight 68.3 ± 13.3 kg, height 170 ± 6 cm) and eight smoking (age 30.5 ± 3.5 yr, weight 60.3 ± 4.9 kg, height 170 ± 6 cm) healthy female volunteers. Smoking women consumed at least 20 cigarettes per day. All subjects showed a normal biphasic pre-treatment cycle and had stopped taking oral contraceptives at least two cycles before entering the study.

2.2 Dosing and sampling

From day 1 to day 21 of the cycle volunteers received one coated tablet of Diane-35® (2 mg CPA, 35 μg EE_2) daily at 8.00 a. m. Venous blood samples were drawn daily at 8.00 a. m. (before intake of the drug) up to the last day of the cycle. Additionally at days 1 and 21 blood was sampled at 0.5, 1, 2, 4, 6, 8, 10 and 12 hours after drug administration.

Blood was immediately centrifuged; plasma was separated and stored at −18°C until analysis.

2.3 Analytic methods

CPA and EE_2 concentration in the plasma were measured by radioimmunoassays after diethylether extraction. CPA-17α-acetoxy-^{3}H (specific activity 0.59 TBq/mmol) and [6,7-^{3}H]-EE_2 (specific activity 1.6 TBq/mmol) were used as tracers. Antisera were raised against CPA-11α-succinoyl-BSA and EE_2-6β-carboxymethyloxime-BSA in rabbits. Details of the procedures are given in references [8, 16].

SHBG and CBG were measured by commercial RIA-kits (Organon Diagnostics, Freiburg (SHBG) and Ire Diagnostics, Düsseldorf (CBG)).

2.4 Evaluation

Terminal half-lives of CPA in the plasma were calculated from the slope of regression line determined from logarithms of concentration for time points ≧ 24 hours after the last administration according to $t_{1/2} = \ln 2/ke$.

Areas under the plasma level curves (AUC_{0-24}) were calculated using the trapezoidal rule.

Extrapolated areas AUC^1_{0-00} after the first administration were calculated from (1) using individual elimination rate constants ke after the last administration.

(1) $AUC^1_{0-00} = AUC^1_{0-24} + C_{24/ke}$.

Accumulation factors were calculated by forming the quotient between the concentrations of CPA 24 hours after the last and the first administration C^{21}_{24}/C^{1}_{24} or between the areas under the CPA plasma level are during day 21 and day 1 $AUC^{21}_{0-24}/AUC^{1}_{0-24}$.

Pharmacokinetic parameters of both treatment groups were compared using the unpaired t-test at $p < 0.05$.

3. Results

3.1 Plasma levels of CPA

Figures 1 and 2 show the concentration of CPA in plasma in non-smoking and in smoking women after the first and last ingestion of Diane-35®.

After the first intake, maximum CPA levels of 16 ± 5 ng/ml and 14 ± 4 ng/ml were found in non-smokers and smokers, respectively, between 1 and 2 hours afters administration. The area under the CPA-plasma level curve during

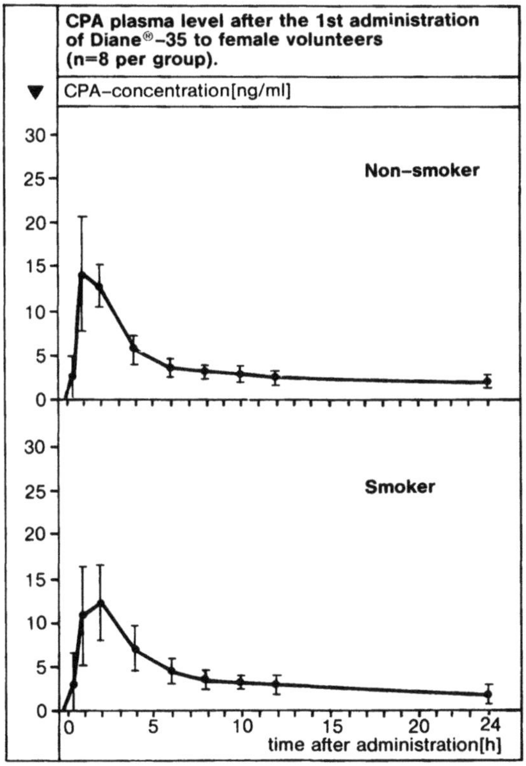

Fig. 1 Time course of the concentration of CPA in the plasma after the 1st administration of Diane-35® to 8 non-smoking (A) and 8 smoking (B) female volunteers. Mean ± SD

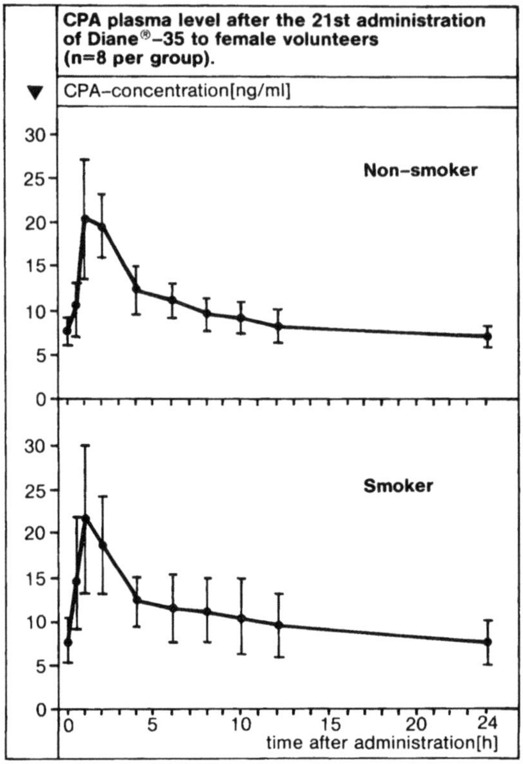

Fig. 2 Time course of the concentration of CPA in the plasma after the 21st administration of Diane-35® to 8 non-smoking (A) and 8 smoking (B) female volunteers. Mean ± SD

the first day (AUC_{0-24}^{1}) was 3.5 ± 0.8 ng × d/ml in non-smokers and 3.9 ± 1.2 ng × d/ml in smokers and increased to AUC_{0-24}^{21}-values of 9.8 ± 1.6 ng × d/ml (non-smokers) and 10.6 ± 3.2 ng × d/ml (smokers) on day 21.

The increase in CPA-plasma levels during a 21-day treatment and the decrease after cessation of intake are given in figure 3 for both treatment groups. Once more, the time courses of CPA-plasma levels were found to be similar in both groups of women. Morning steady-state plasma levels (C_{min}^{ss}) of 6—8 ng/ml were reached after, at least, 10 administrations.

After the last ingestion, CPA concentrations decayed with a terminal half-life of 4.2 ± 1.8 days (non-smokers) and 3.5 ± 1.0 day (smokers).

From a comparison of the corresponding CPA-concentrations 24 hours after the 21st and after the first administration, a mean accumulation factor of 4.3 was calculated for smokers and non-smokers (tab. 1). From the quotient of AUC-values ($AUC_{0-24}^{21}/AUC_{0-24}^{1}$) an accumulation factor of 2.9 was derived for both groups.

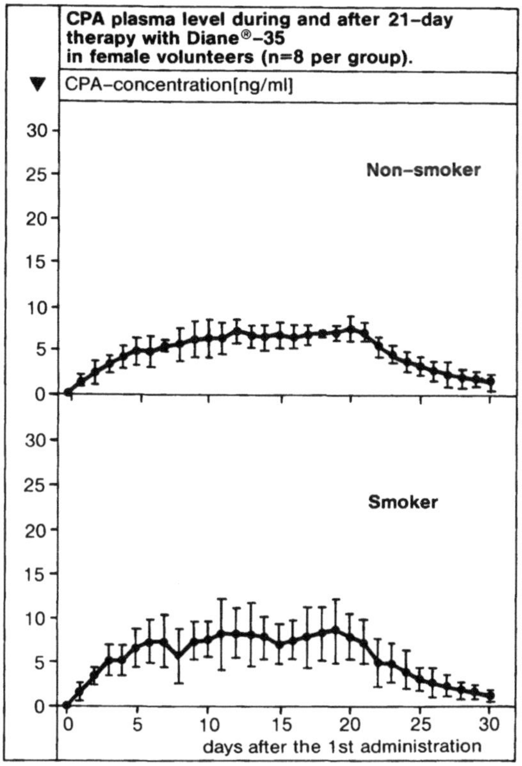

Fig. 3 Time course of the concentration of CPA in the plasma ($C_{24\,h}$) in 8 non-smoking (A) and 8 smoking (B) female volunteers during and after 21-day treatment with Diane-35®. Mean ± SD

3.2 Plasma levels of EE_2

Plasma levels of EE_2 exceeded the detection limit of 40 pg/ml only between 0.5 and 8 hours after administration.

In non-smoking women the maximum concentration of EE_2 in the plasma of 0.10 ± 0.04 ng/ml (day 1) and 0.12 ± 0.03 ng/ml (day 21) were reached 1.3 ± 0.5 hours after administration. Areas under the plasma level time curve were 0.50 ± 0.11 ng × h/ml (day 1) and 0.54 ± 0.31 ng × h/ml (day 21) respectively. In smoking women maximum EE_2-values of 0.09 ± 0.04 ng/ml (day 1) and of 0.15 ± 0.07 ng/ml (day 21) were measured 2.1 ± 1.3 h and 2.6 ± 2.7 h after the intake. The corresponding AUC-values were calculated to be 0.65 ± 0.57 ng × h/ml and 1.7 ± 1.5 ng × h/ml (tab. 1).

No differences in pharmacokinetic parameters (C_{max}, t_{max}, AUC) of EE_2 between non-smoking and smoking women were found either after the first or after the 21st administration.

Table 1 Pharmacokinetic parameters calculated from CPA and EE_2 plasma levels after single and repeated daily oral administration of Diane 35 to 8 non-smoking (NS) and 8 smoking (S) women. Means ± s.d.

	NS	S	NS	S
	CPA		EE_2	
1st administration				
C^1_{max} (ng/ml)	16±5	14±4	0.10±0.04	0.09±0.04
C^1_{24} (ng/ml)	1.6±0.7	1.9±0.8	–	–
t_{max} (h)	1.4±0.5	1.8±1.0	1.3 ±0.5	2.1 ±1.3
AUC^1_{0-24}	3.5±0.8*	3.9±1.2*	0.50±0.11**	0.65±0.57**
AUC^1_{0-00}	12.8±4.8*	14.2±5.4*	0.50±0.11**	0.65±0.57**
21st administration				
C^{21}_{max} (ng/ml)	22±5	24±5	0.12±0.03	0.15±0.07
C^{21}_{24} (ng/ml)	7.1±1.2	7.4±2.7	–	–
t_{max} (h)	1.3±0.5	1.9±2.5	1.3 ±0.5	2.6 ±2.7
$t_{1/2}$ term. (d)	4.2±1.8	3.5±1.0	–	–
AUC^{21}_{0-24}	9.8±1.6*	10.6±3.2*	0.54±0.31**	1.7 ±1.5*
Accumulation factor:				
$R = C^{21}_{24}/C^1_{24}$	4.3±1.3	4.3±1.0	–	–
$R = AUC^{21}_{0-24}/AUC^1_{0-24}$	2.9±0.6	2.9±0.9	–	–

* AUCs for CPA are given in ng × d/ml
** AUCs for EE_2 are given in ng × h/ml

3.3 Plasma levels of SHBG

The concentrations of SHBG increased during 21 days of treatment with Diane-35® from an initial level of 47 ± 23 nmol/l to 178 ± 57 nmol/l in non-smoking women and from 51 ± 21 nmol/l to 176 ± 63 nmol/l in smoking women (fig. 4). Within 10 days after the last administration, the concentration of SHBG decreased in both groups but did not return to the initial levels.

3.4 Plasma levels of CBG

The level of CBG in the plasma at the beginning of the cycle was 40 ± 6 µg/ml in non-smoking women and 37 ± 5 µg/ml in smoking women. The concentration of CGB increased during treatment with Diane-35® to levels of 76 ± 7 µg/ml in non-smoking women and 77 ± 9 µg/ml in smoking women. After the last administration, the CBG concentration decreased in both groups and reached plasma levels of 56 ± 6 µg/ml and 51 ± 9 µg/ml, respectively, on day 30. No difference in CBG levels was seen between non-smoking and smoking women (fig. 5).

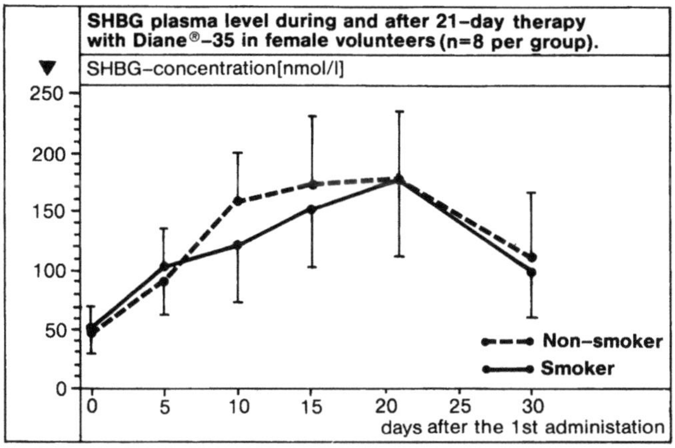

Fig. 4 Time course of the concentration of SHBG in the plasma in 8 non-smoking and 8 smoking female volunteers during and after 21-day treatment with Diane-35®.

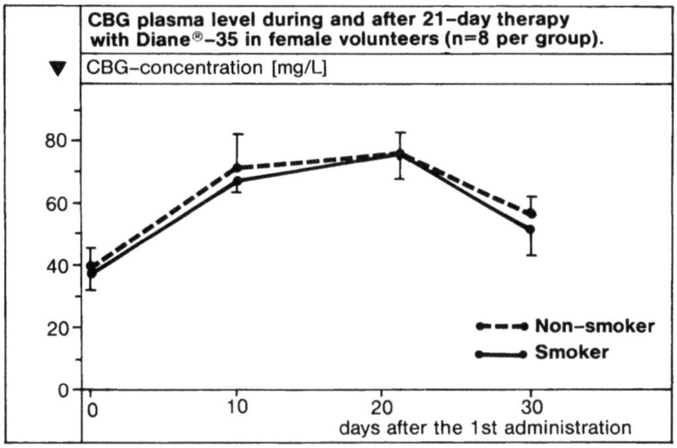

Fig. 5 Time course of the concentration of CBG in the plasma in 8 non-smoking and 8 smoking female volunteers during and after 21-day treatment with Diane-35®.

4. Discussion

The pharmacokinetic behaviour of CPA after single and multiple administration of Diane-35® was similar to that of Diane-50® [3]. CPA was rapidly absorbed and completely bioavailable as indicated by C_{max}-values of 16 ± 5 ng/ml (non-smokers) and 14 ± 4 ng/ml and AUC_{0-24}-values of 3.5 ± 0.8 ng × d/ml (non-smokers) and 3.9 ± 1.2 ng × d/ml (smokers). Düsterberg et al. [3] reported maximum CPA levels of 11.0 ± 3.4 ng/ml and AUC_{0-24}-values of 3.3

± 1.3 ng × d/ml after a single dose of Diane-50®. In the present study the terminal half-life after cessation of treatment was 4.2 ± 1.8 days in non-smokers and 3.5 ± 1.0 days in smokers. After a 21-day treatment with Diane-50® a terminal half-life of 2.9 ± 0.7 days was found [3]. The somewhat longer- half-lives found in the present study can be explained by the longer follow-up of plasma levels (up to 10 days after the last administration). Binding experiments with ^{3}H-testosterone and ^{3}H-dihydrotestosterone did not show any influence of CPA on binding of ligands to SHBG [5]. Obviously CPA is not bound to SHBG and a 3-fold increase of SHBG levels during therapy with Diane-35® does not alter CPA-phamacokinetics.

The variance of the accumulation factors calculated (2.9 and 4.3) was dependent on the method used for determination. The factor of 2.9, which was obtained by a comparison of areas, seems to be the more stable method and agrees with the ratio of 2.4 ± 0.7 reported by Düsterberg et al. [3].

EE_2 plasma levels after oral administration of Diane-35® were rather low and showed a considerable scatter, especially in the groups of smoking women. Peak levels of approximately 0.1 ng/ml, found between 1 and 2 hours, corresponded to the 2.5-fold detection limit. Maximum levels in the present study were of the same magnitude as those reported after administration of Diane-50® (0,08 ± 0.03 ng/ml). Because of this high inter-subject variability in the bioavailability of EE_2 and the low absolute EE_2-levels [8], it was not possible to discriminate a dose difference of 15 μg EE_2 between Diane-35® and Diane-50®.

The concentration of SHBG and CBG in the plasma can be used as an indicator for the "total estrogenicity" of an oral contraceptive preparation [10, 17, 18]. Estrogens increase the total circulating SHBG and CBG in the plasma, while progestogens with androgenic partial effects antagonize estrogen induced synthesis of SHBG [10, 17].

Twenty-one day treatment with Diane-35® led to plateau levels of CBG and SHBG which were approximately 2 to 3 times higher than initial levels at the beginning of the cycle. This confirms that CPA is an antiandrogen with progestogenic activity but without androgenicity.

After the intake-free period pre-treatment levels of CBG and SHBG were not reaches. It has been documented that even a 2 week estrogen-free period is not sufficient for return of elevated levels to normal [17]. Increased SHBG plasma levels lead to decreased free testosterone levels, an effect which may contribute to the good therapeutic effect of Diane in the treatment on androgenic symptoms in women.

The treatment of both a group of non-smoking and a group of smoking women with Diane-35® did not indicate any differences in either the pharmacokinetics of CPA and EE_2 or the effect on plasma levels of CBG and SHBG. Obviously, the induction of drug metabolising enzymes by tobacco smoke, which is more extensive in young than in older subjects [19, 21], does not influence the bioavailability of EE_2 and CPA. Consequently, an equal therapeutic effect of Diane-35® treatment in non-smoking and smoking women may be anticipated.

5. Summary

Cyproterone acetate (CPA) and ethinyl estradiol (EE_2) plasma levels were followed during day 1 and day 21 of daily treatment with Diane-35® in two groups of 8 non-smoking and 8 smoking women. Additionally, CPA, sex hormone binding globulin (SHBG), and corticosteroid binding globulin (CBG) plasma concentrations were measured during and after cessation of therapy.

CPA and EE_2 are rapidly and completely absorbed after oral administration of Diane-35®. Due to its relatively long terminal half-life (3—4 days), CPA accumulates during the 21 day treatment by a factor of approximately 3—4. No accumulation was observed for EE_2. SHBG- and CBG-plasma levels on day 21 were 3- and 2-times above initial levels on day 1.

There was no difference between non-smoking and smoking women found in any parameter investigated.

References

[1] Becker, H., B. Düsterberg, H. Klosterhalfen: Bioavailability of cyproterone acetate after oral and intramuscular application in men. Urol. Int. **35** (1980) 381—385.

[2] Beckett, A. H., E. J. Triggs: Enzyme induction in man caused by smoking. Nature (London) **216** (1967) 587—588.

[3] Daniel, S.: Die Pharmakokinetik von Cyproteronacetat unter der hochdosierten oralen Standardtherapie bei androgenisierten Frauen. Thesis, Free University of Berlin, Medical Faculty, 1985.

[4] Düsterberg, B., M. Hümpel, H. Wendt: Plasma levels of active ingredients after single and repeated administration of a new oral contraceptive containing 2 mg cyproterone acetate and 50 µg of ethinyl estradiol (Diane®) to five young women. Acta Obstet. Gynecol. Scand. Suppl. **88** (1979) 27—31.

[5] Frölich, M., M. G. Vanschie, E. C. Brand: Sex hormone binding globulins: Binding capacity and studies on the binding of cyproterone acetate and other steroids. Clin. Chim. Acta **87** (1978) 239—244.

[6] Hammerstein, J., J. Meckies, I. Leo-Rossberg et al.: Use of cyproterone acetate in the treatment of acne, hirsutism and virilism. J. Steroid. Biochem. **6** (1975) 827.

[7] Hümpel, M., G. Dogs, H. Wendt et al.: Plasmaspiegel und Pharmakokinetik von Cyproteronacetat nach oraler Applikation als 50-mg-Tablette bei 5 Männern. Drug. Res. **28** (1978) 319—322.

[8] Hümpel, M., B. Nieuweboer, H. Wendt et al.: Investigations of pharmacokinetics of ethinyl-estradiol to specific consideration of a possible first pass effect in women. Contraception **19** (1979) 421—432.

[9] Hümpel, M., H. Wendt, P. E. Schulze et al.: Bioavailability and pharmacokinetics of 2.0 mg cyproterone acetate in combination with 50 μg ethinyl estradiol to 6 young women. Contraception **15** (1977) 579—588.
[10] Jusko, W. J.: Role of tobacco smoking in pharmacokinetics. J. Pharmacokinet. Biopharm. **6** (1978) 7—39.
[11] Kammen, E. van, J. H. H. Thikssen, B. Rodenaker et al.: The influence of hormonal contraceptives on sex hormon binding globulin (SHBG) capacity. Contraception **11** (1975) 53—59.
[12] Moltz, L., J. Mechies, J. Hammerstein: Die klinische Anwendung von Antiandrogenen bei der Frau. Gynäkologie **13** (1980) 1—17.
[13] Moltz, L., J. Meckies, J. Hammerstein: Die kontrazeptive Bedeutung androgenisierter Frauen mit einem niedrig dosierten cyproteronacetathaltigen Einphasenpräparat. Dtsch. Med. Wochenschr. **194** (1979) 1376.
[14] Neumann, F.: Klinik der Antiandrogene. D. Ärzteblatt **75** (1978) 1633.
[15] Neumann, F., A. Schleusner, M. Hümpel: Antiandrogene—Pharmakologische Grundlagen—. Der Gynäkologe **12** (1979) 228—242.
[16] Nieuweboer, B., K. Lübke: Radioimmunological determination of cyproterone acetate. Horm. Res. **8** (1977) 210.
[17] Schwartz, U., J. Hammerstein: The oestrogenic potency of various contraceptive steroids as determined by their effects on transcortin-binding capacity. Acta Endocrin. **76** (1974) 159—1781.
[18] Trienekens, P. H., N. A. Schmidt, J. H. H. Thijssen: The effect of age, weight related parameters and hormonal contraceptives on androgenical assays. Contraception **33** (1986) 503—517.
[19] Vestal, R. W., A. H. Norris, J. D. Tobin et al.: Antipyrine metabolism in man: influence of age, alcohol, caffeine and smoking. Clin. Pharmacol. Ther. **18** (1975) 425—432.
[20] Welch, R. M., Y. E. Harrison, B. W. Gommi et al.: Stimulatory effects of cigarette smoking on the hydroxylation of 3,4-benzpyrene and the N-demethylation of 3-methyl-4-monomethylamino benzene on enzymes in human placenta. Clin. Pharmacol. Ther. **10** (1969) 100—109.
[21] Wood, A. J. J., R. E. Vestal, G. R. Wilkinson et al.: Effect of aging and cigarette smoking on antipyrine and indocyanine green elimination. Clin. Pharmacol. Ther. **26** (1979) 16—20.

Ovulation inhibitory effect of SH B 209 AE (Diane-35®)—a new antiandrogen-estrogen combination

J. Spona, J. Huber, J. B. Schmidt

Introduction

The antiandrogen action of cyproterone acetate (CPA) is well documented. In addition, cyproterone acetate was found to have the biological activity of a progestagen when given orally [2]. Several lines of evidence suggest that cyproterone acetate is biologically more active as progestagen than chlormadinone acetate or medroxyprogesterone acetate [6]. Furthermore, cyproterone acetate elicits a greater antiandrogen action than either chlormadinone acetate or medroxyprogesterone acetate. Cyproterone acetate was therefore used in combination with ethinyl estradiol for the therapy of androgenisation in the female [5]. Until recently the therapy was performed by using a combined preparation containing 2 mg cyproterone acetate and 50 µg ethinyl estradiol. Good therapy results were obtained in patients suffering from seborrhea, acne, and alopecia androgenetica [12]. In subjects with severe androgenizations, a high-dose cyproterone acetate therapy can be used [5].

The aim of the present investigation was to determine the lowest dose of cyproterone acetate which assures inhibition of ovulation (borderline dose) and to investigate the efficacy for inhibition of ovulation of 2 mg cyproterone acetate in combination with 35 µg ethinyl estradiol. The study was aimed at complying with the suggestion of the WHO [15] to use the lowest possible dose resulting in a therapy.

Materials and methods

The borderline dose of cyproterone acetate was studied in 12 volunteers, aged 20 to 28 years, who had normal ovulatory cycles. Subjects were monitored during one control cycle and during one treatment cycle. During the treatment cycle subjects were treated orally with 0.125, 0.25, 0.50, or 1.0 mg of cyproterone acetate from day 5 through day 25 of their cycles. LH, FSH, 17β-estradiol and progesterone were estimated daily from day 5 of the cycle. Additionally, cervical score and karyopycnotic index were registered.

The efficacy of a combination of 2 mg cyproterone acetate and 35 μg ethinyl estradiol was studied in 6 female volunteers who had normal cycles. The treatment was started on day 5 and discontinued on day 25. Subjects were monitored by daily estimation of LH, FSH, 17β-estradiol, progesterone, testosterone, prolactin, and SHBG. Cervical score and karyopycnotic index were determined. In addition, antithrombin III was estimated during the first and the third treatment cycle. Blood samples were taken between 8 and 9 a.m.

Radioimmunoassay of 17β-estradiol and progesterone was carried out with solid phase methods [3] using materials obtained from Diagnostic Products Corporation (Los Angeles, CA 90045, USA). The assay of prolactin, FSH, and SHBG was carried out with reagents from Serono Diagnostic S.A. (Centre Industriel, CH-Coinsins, Switzerland). Radioimmunoassay of LH and testosterone was performed with reagents obtained from Sorin, Biomedica, S.P.A (13040 Saluggia, Italy). Antithrombin III was determined with method of Coattest Antithrombin Kabi Vitrum (Kabi Vitrum, A-1232 Wien, Austria).

The intraassay and interassay coefficients of variation varied between 7% and 12%. Statistical analyses of hormone serum levels were performed with variance analyses.

Results

The determination of borderline doses of ovulation inhibition by cyproterone acetate showed that 2/5 of the subjects exhibited normal cycles at a 0.5 mg dose. 3/5 of the subjects showed inhibition of ovulation with follicular maturation (tab. 1). 5/5 of the subjects exhibited inhibition of ovulation when treated with 1.0 mg cyproterone acetate and 4/5 of the subjects showed follicular maturation. This data (tab. 1) suggests that the borderline dose for inhibition of ovulation is 1 mg cyproterone acetate.

In order to obtain a good antiandrogen efficacy, 2 mg cyproterone acetate were combined with 35 μg ethinyl estradiol. Inhibition of ovulation with this combined preparation was also investigated. Serum levels of LH and FSH during the control cycle and during the first and third therapy cycles are shown in figure 1. All females exhibited normal control cycles. Inhibition of ovulation was noted during treatment cycles. A decrease of LH and FSH serum levels during days 5 through 25 of the treatment cycles is noteworthy (fig. 1). Patterns of progesterone serum levels (fig. 2) are suggestive of anovulatory cycles.

Patterns of 17β-estradiol serum levels (fig. 2) suggest normal follicular maturation during the control cycle and suppression of follicular maturation during the first treatment cycle. On the other hand, the patterns observed suggested follicular maturation during the third treatment cycle (fig. 2). Data shown in fi-

Table 1 Borderline dose for inhibition of ovulation by cyproterone acetate in 12 volunteers.

Cyproterone acetate					
Dose (μg/day)	n	Inhibition of ovulation	with follicular maturation	luteal-insufficiency	normal cycle
0.125	1	–	–	–	1
0.25	1	–	–	–	1
0.50	5	3	3	–	2
1.00	5	5	4	–	–

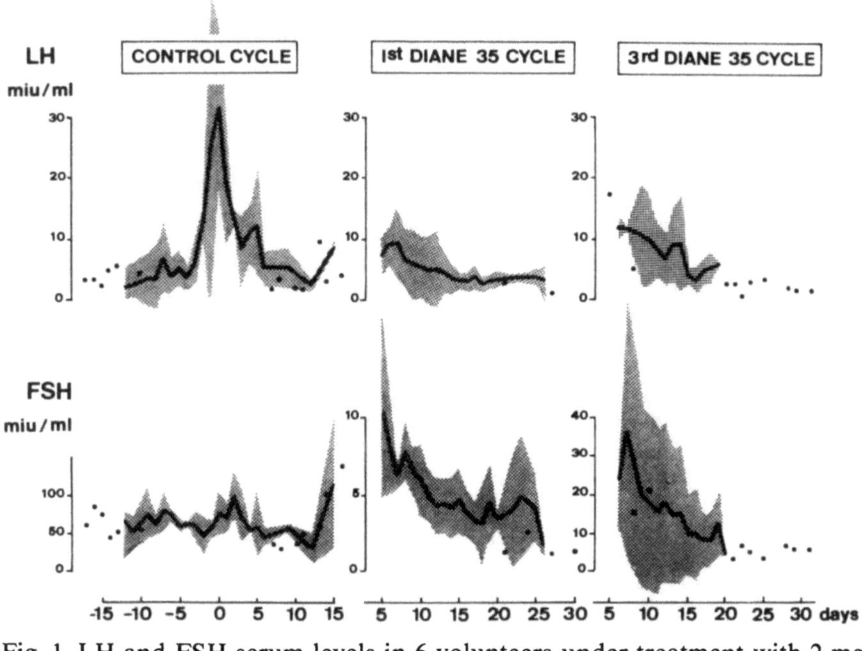

Fig. 1 LH and FSH serum levels in 6 volunteers under treatment with 2 mg cyproterone acetate and 35 μg ethinyl estradiol. Control cycle (C), first cycle (I), third cycle (III).

gures 1 and 2 are means ± SD obtained from 6 females. Analyses of individual cycles indicated that one female presented with follicular maturation during the third treatment cycle (fig. 3). This data on estradiol serum levels during the third treatment cycle resulted in patterns of combined data of figure 2. It is noteworthy that the female presenting with high 17β-estradiol serum levels during the third treatment cycle also showed a slight increase of 17β-estradiol serum levels during days 5 to 10 in the first treatment cycle (fig. 3). On the other hand, a deacrease of LH and FSH was noted in this subject during the third treatment cycle (fig. 4).

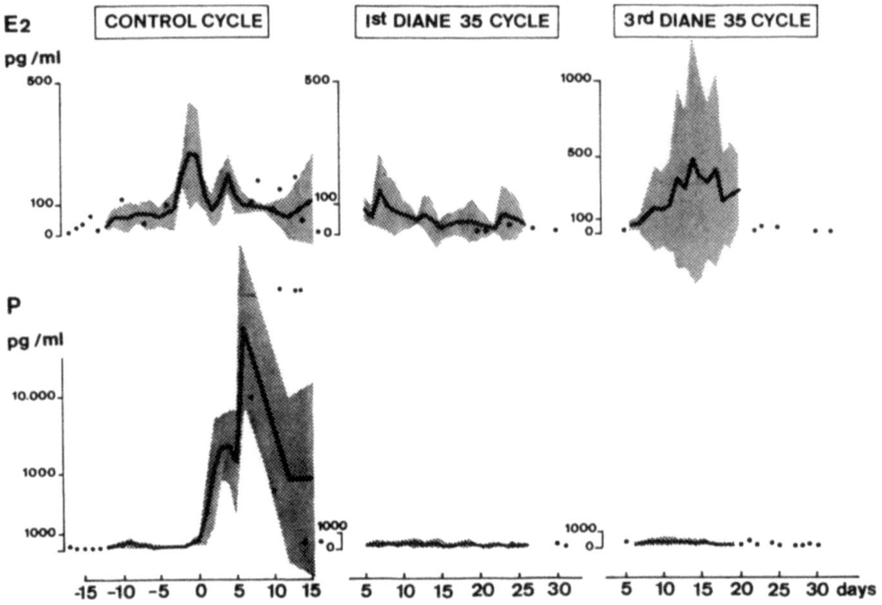

Fig. 2 17β-estradiol (E_2) and progesterone (P) serum levels in 6 females under treatment with 2 mg cyproterone acetate and 35 μg ethinyl estradiol. Control cycle (C), first cycle (I), third cycle (III).

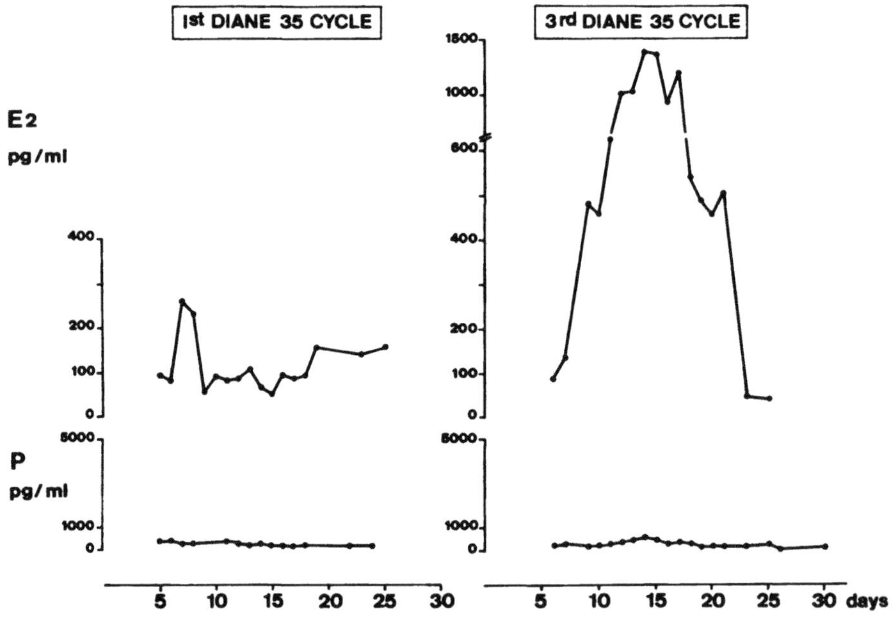

Fig. 3 17β-estradiol (E_2) and progesterone serum levels in one female under treatment with 2 mg cyproterone acetate and 35 μg ethinyl estradiol. First cycle (I), third cycle (III).

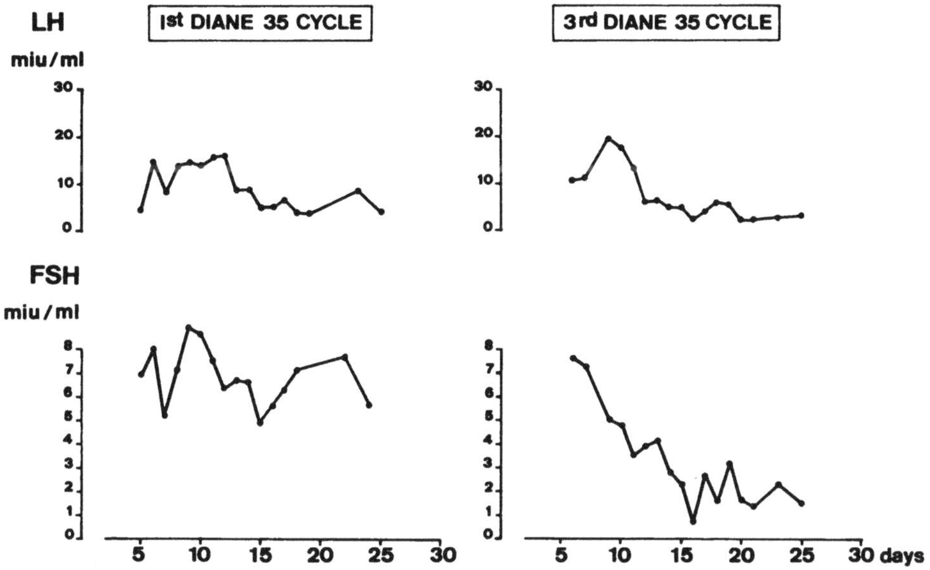

Fig. 4 LH and FSH serum levels under treatment with 2 mg cyproterone acetate and 35 µg ethinyl estradiol in one female. First cycle (I), third cycle (III).

Statistical analyses of LH and FSH serum levels (tab. 2) shows that the gonadotropins are significantly suppressed during the first treatment cycle. A significant difference of FSH serum levels between the first and third therapy cycle with 2 mg cyproterone acetate and 35 µg ethinyl estradiol was noted (tab. 2). Progesterone serum levels and 17β-estradiol serum levels during the control cycle were significantly different from first therapy cycle ($p < 0.0025$ and $p < 0.05$). Progesterone serum levels did not show a significant difference between the first and third therapy cycle, whereas for 17β-estradiol serum levels significant differences between the first and third therapy cycle ($p < 0.005$) were found.

Additionally, changes in SHBG, testosterone and prolactin serum levels during therapy are of interest (tab. 3). During the treatment with 2 mg cyproterone

Table 2 LH and FSH serum levels under treatment with 2 mg cyproterone acetate and 35 µg ethinyl estradiol in 6 females. Control cycle (C), first cycle (I) and third cycle (III). Data given as means ± SD. N.s. = Not significant.

	C	I	III
LH (mIU/ml)	7.45 ±7.16	4.17±2.30	5.89±4.22
FSH (mIU/ml)	6.554±2.01	4.81±1.86	6.55±3.28

	C vs. I	C vs. III	I vs. III
LH (mIU/ml)	$p < 0.05$	n.s.	n.s.
FSH (mIU/ml	$p < 0.0005$	n.s.	$p < 0.01$

Table 3 SHBG, testosterone and prolactin serum levels under treatment with 2 mg cyproterone acetate and 35 μg ethinyl estradiol in 6 volunteers. Control cycle (C), first cycle (I), third cycle (III). Data are given as means ± SD. N.s. = not significant.

	C	I	III
SHBG (μg %)	2.77±0.54	4.26±0.92	4.85±0.49
T (ng/ml)	0.32±0.17	0.22±0.08	0.37±0.14
hPRL (ng/ml)	10.05±4.62	11.49±6.00	12.59±5.49

	C vs. I	C vs. III	I vs. III
SHBG (μg %)	$p < 0.0005$	$p < 0.0005$	$p < 0.0125$
T (ng/ml)	$p < 0.005$	n.s.	$p < 0.005$
hPRL (ng/ml)	n.s.	$p < 0.05$	n.s.

acetate in combination with 35 μg ethinyl estradiol a significant increase of SHBG serum levels during the first treatment cycle was noted. A further increase of SHBG serum levels during the third treatment cycle was also observed (tab. 3). On the other hand, while treatment with this oral contraceptive resulted in inhibition of testosterone serum levels during the first treatment cycle, no significant difference of testosterone serum levels was noted between the third therapy cycle and control cycle (tab. 3). Treatment resulted in a slight increase of prolactin serum levels (tab. 3), which, although significantly higher in the third treatment cycle than during the control cycle, remained within the normal range. Therapy with this combination did not result in changes of antithrombine III.

Discussion

It is well documented that cyproterone acetate exhibits competitive binding with the androgen receptor. This results in good therapeutic effects of this antiandrogen in patients with seborrhea, acne, hirsutism and alopecia androgenetica. In patients with androgenization, both increased androgen serum levels and a greater end-organ sensitivity to androgens may cause androgenization. Use of antiandrogens for the treatment of acne was described [1] after the progestagen action of cyproterone acetate had been reported [2]. Until recently a combination of 2 mg cyproterone acetate with 50 μg ethinyl estradiol was used. Present data show that the borderline dose for effective inhibition of ovulation with cyproterone acetate is 1 mg per day. The efficacy of low-dose oral cyproterone acetate therapy is well documented in patients with mild androgenization. It was noted that patients with medium forms of hirsutism and severe acne benefit most by combining the low-dose regimen containing 2 mg cyproterone acetate plus 50 μg ethinyl estradiol with an additional dose of cyproterone acetate [13]. Indications for antiandrogen therapy using the combined preparation of oral contraceptives have been described [16]. Recent studies indicate that the application of a combined preparation containing cyproterone acetate and ethinyl estradiol results in a 60% reduction of acne within 6 months and a 30% reduction of the sebum excretion rate within 3 months [4, 10].

A reduction of the estrogen dose from 50 µg to 35 µg in a combination preparation with 2 mg cyproterone acetate was investigated in the present study in order to comply with WHO suggestion [15] that no more than the minimum effective dose be used. Results of the present investigation show that a combination of 2 mg cyproterone acetate with 35 µg ethinyl estradiol results in inhibition of ovulation in all subjects. Follicular maturation in one female during the third treatment cycle is in line with other reports on this phenomenon during treatment with low-dose oral contraceptives. It is noteworthy that the treatment with 2 mg cyproterone acetate and 35 µg ethinyl estradiol resulted in a severe suppression of FSH serum levels which rose during the tablet-free interval between treatment cycles. Suppression of FSH serum levels caused an arrest of follicular maturation in 5/6 females. On the other hand, this low-dose oral contraceptive resulted in complete inhibition of cervical score and suppression of karyopycnotic index.

Additionally, the stimulation of SHBG serum concentration during the first and third treatment cycle with 2 mg cyproterone acetate and 35 µg ethinyl estradiol tends to support the expectation that this new oral contraceptive should exhibit similar efficacy for the therapy of androgenization as does the one with the higher estrogen dose [9, 11]. Furthermore, a reduction of total testosterone during the first treatment cycle adds to the blunting of free testosterone concentration in the serum. In addition, it is of interest that the application of this new oral contraceptive does not result in pathological changes of antithrombine III and prolactin serum levels.

The development of an oral contraceptive containing an antiandrogen [8] allowed the treatment of signs of androgenization in the female such as acne, seborrhea, and hirsutism with cyproterone acetate [7, 14]. Present data combine to suggest that the reduction of the estrogen dose from 50 µg to 35 µg per day in combination preparations with 2 mg cyproterone acetate does not affect complete inhibition of ovulation.

References

[1] Fanta, D., W. H. F. Schneider, J. Spona et al.: Die Anwendung von Antiandrogenen in der Behandlung der Akne. Wien. klin. Wschr. **89** (1977) 622—624.

[2] Fixson, U.: Vorläufige Mitteilung über ein neues oral wirksames Gestagen. Geburtsh. u. Frauenheilk. **23** (1963) 371—376.

[3] Gitsch, E., W. H. F. Schneider, J. Spona: Der Radioimmunoassay. In: Gitsch, E. (ed.): Radioisotope in Geburtshilfe und Frauenheilkunde, pp. 373. Walter de Gruyter, Berlin 1977.
[4] Greenwood, R., B. Burke, L. Brummitt et al.: Cyclic Cyproterone/Ethinylestradiol for Acne. Lancet **1** (1983) 796.
[5] Hammerstein, J., B. Cupceanu: Die Behandlung des Hirsutismus mit CPA. Dtsch. med. Wsch. **94** (1969) 829—833.
[6] Kauffmann, C.: Umwandlung der Uterusschleimhaut einer kastrierten Frau aus dem atrophischen Stadium in das der sekretorischen Funktion durch Ovarialhormone. Zbl. Gynäk. **34** (1932) 2058—2061.
[7] Keller, J. P., A. Fetz, A. Schär et al.: Behandlung von Akne Seborrhö mit Antiandrogenen. Schweiz. Med. Wsch. **108** (1978) 1640—1644.
[8] Lachnit-Fixson, U.: The Development and Evaluation of an Ovulation Inhibitor (Diane) Containing an Antiandrogen. Acta Obstet. Gynecol. Scand. Suppl. **88** (1979) 33—37.
[9] Ludwig, E., W. Meinhof, H. Zaun: Zur Therapie androgenabhängiger Hauterscheinungen mit Cyproteronacetat-Östrogen-Kombination. Aktuelle Dermatol. **3** (1977) 32—36.
[10] Marsden, J., S. Shuster: Cyclic Cyproterone/Ethinylestradiol for Acne. Lancet **1** (1983) 736.
[11] Moltz, L., J. Meckies, J. Hammerstein: Die kontrazeptive Betreuung androgenisierter Frauen mit einem niedrig dosierten cyproteronacetathaltigen Einphasenpräparat. Dtsch. med. Wschr. **104** (1979) 1376—1381.
[12] Moltz, L., U. Schwartz, J. Hammerstein: Klinische Anwendungen von Antiandrogenen bei der Frau. Gynäkologe **13** (1980) 1—6.
[13] Moltz, E., E. Kaiser: Mittelhochdosierte orale Cyproteronacetat-Therapie bei Frauen mit mittelgradig ausgeprägten Androgenisierungserscheinungen. Ergebnisse einer multizentrischen Doppelblind-Studie. Geburtsh. u. Frauenheilk. **44** (1984) 47—51.
[14] Taubert, H. D., O. Jürgensen: Die Behandlung des Hirsutismus und anderer Störungen des Haarfollikelapparates mit Antiandrogenen. Therapiewoche **28** (1978) 2951—2956.
[15] WHO — World Health Organization: Steroid contraception and the risk of neoplasia. WHO Tech. Rep. Ser. (1978) 619.
[16] Zaun, H., E. Ludwig: Dermatologische Indikationsstellung zur antiandrogenen Behandlung. Zeitschr. f. Hautkrankh. **53** (1978) 759—764.

A study to investigate the maintenance of ovulation inhibition when patients switch over from Diane to Diane-35®

H. P. Higgins, T. G. Davies, P. E. Hutchinson

Introduction

50 microgram ethinyl estradiol plus 2 milligram cyproterone acetate (Diane) has been found to be effective in treating severe acne in females, producing a 74% improvement in clinical grading of acne and a 25% decrease in sebum secretion rate [1—3]. In addition Diane provides contraceptive cover which is of the same order of efficacy as any currently available combined oral contraceptive.

More recently a lower dose formulation, 35 microgram ethinyl estradiol / 2 milligram cyproterone acetate (Diane-35®) has been produced. This preparation has been shown to have equal efficacy to the higher dose ethinyl estradiol preparation in terms of the treatment of acne vulgaris [4]. This preparation has also been shown to be as effective a contraceptive as the higher estrogen preparation.

It is likely that Clinicians may wish to change patients from Diane to Diane-35®. The aim of the present study was to determine whether contraceptive cover continues uninterrupted on change of preparation. Two dosage schedules were considered, first the low dose preparation starting on day 1 of the ensuing cycle, and second there being a 7 day interval between the two preparations.

Method

Theoretical considerations

The presence or absence of ovulation has been investigated indirectly via estradiol, progesterone, FSH and LH changes through the menstrual cycle.

The familiar, expected, normal pattern of change of ovarian steroid hormones during the ovulatory menstrual cycle is shown in figure 1. The serum progesterone rises after ovulation, being produced in large amounts by the cor-

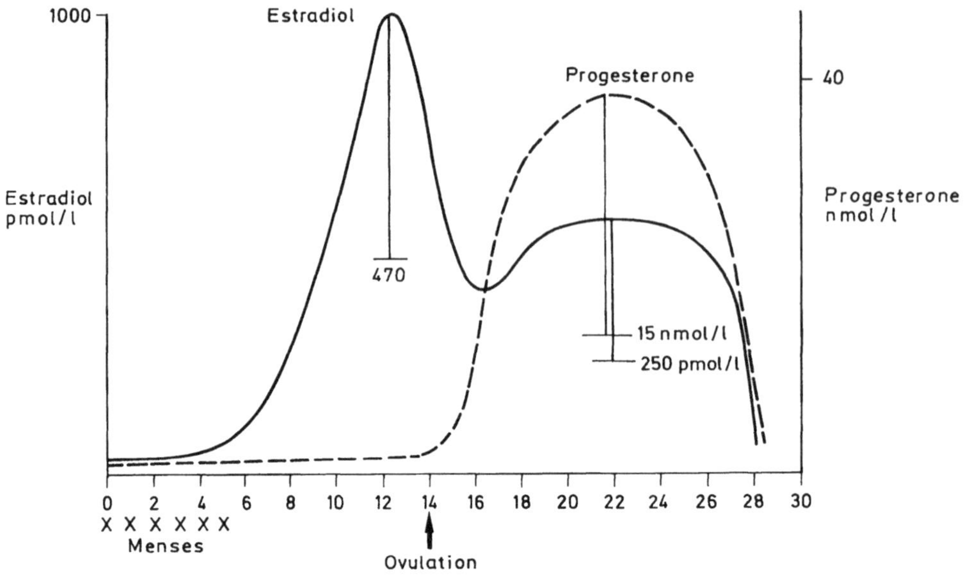

Fig. 1 Ovarian steroid cycles related to a 28 day menstrual cycle

pus luteum, from a basal follicular level of approximately 2 nmol/l to a peak of approximately 40 nmol/l. Estradiol has a biphasic pattern, with a large pre-ovulatory peak of approximately 1,000 pmol/l, and a more steady rise during the luteal phase to approximately 500 pmol/l, the basal levels being of the order of 50—100 pmol/l. For the purpose of the present study, the lower limits of these peak values compatible with a normal ovulatory cycle, the "minimal ovulatory levels" (M.O.L.), have been taken as: —for the peak luteal progesterone—15 nmol/l, pre-ovulatory peak estradiol—470 pmol/l and peak luteal estradiol—250 pmol/l.

Considering the gonadotrophins (fig. 2) there is a peak of both LH and FSH, which occurs over a narrow, 2 day, interval at the time of ovulation. The ovulatory urinary M.O.L. for LH is of the order of 7 IU/mmol creatinine.

In women taking oral contraceptives these hormonal peaks are suppressed. The present data were analysed basically in two ways. The first was an external comparison of observed peak levels with the respective M.O.L.'s. The second was an internal comparison of observed peak levels with observed basal levels. Failure to demonstrate any differences between these would suggest complete suppression of the hormone cycles.

Patients and methods

13 patients took part in the study. These were female patients aged between 16—30 years, in whom there were none of the accepted contra-indications for

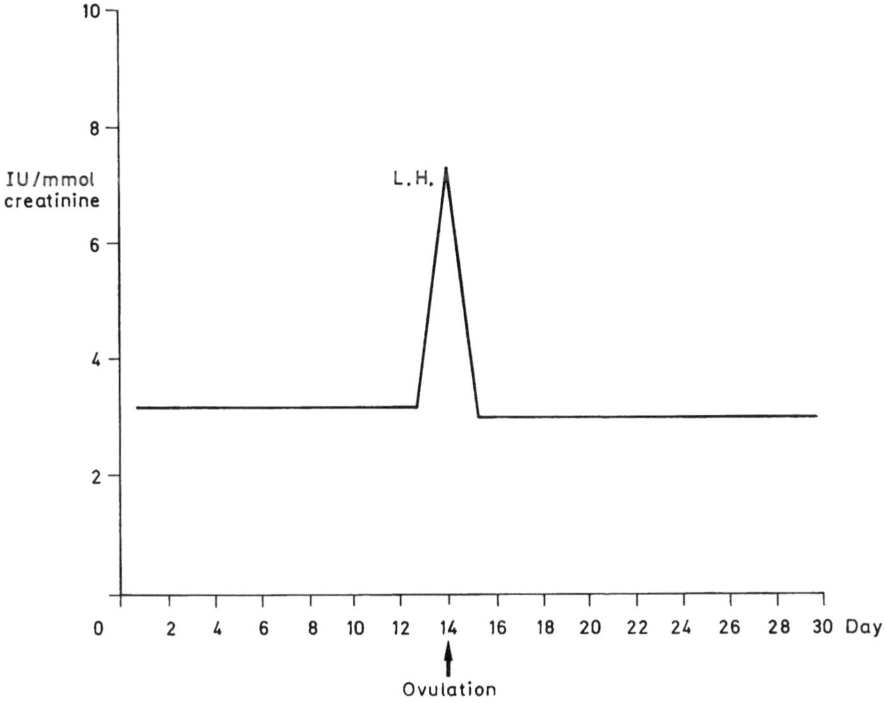

Fig. 2 Gonadotrophin cycle related to a 28 day menstrual cycle

oral contraceptives and who had been taking Diane as treatment for acne vulgaris for at least three cycles preceding entry into the study. None of the patients was lactating nor was taking systemic therapy.

The patients were divided into two groups, "A" and "B", on a random basis. In Group "A" there was a time interval of 7 days following the last Diane-50® tablet prior to taking the Diane-35®. In Group "B" there was no similar time interval and patients took the Diane-35® on the first day of the subsequent menstrual loss.

The radioimmunoassay systems of Coat A Count (Diagnostic Products Corporation), Sorin and the Chelsea Hospital were used to estimate the levels respectively of progesterone, estradiol and the gonadotrophins.

For the ovarian steroid estimations, blood was taken on one day between days 0—4, 5—7, 8—11, 12—14, 15—17, and 18—21. The peak luteal progesterone level was taken as that obtained between days 18—21. The mean follicular level was the arithmetic mean of all levels obtained between days 1—14 in each individual. The peak luteal estradiol level was similarly taken as that level obtained between days 18—21. The pre-ovulatory peak estrogen level was taken as the highest value in each individual of the levels obtained between days 10—14. The basal estrogen level was taken as the level obtained between days 1—4.

For the gonadotrophin estimations, early morning specimens of urine were taken on each of days 12—17. The advantages of this method of sampling, which required small samples taken over a fairly protracted period, are first that there is a high chance of striking any true ovulatory gonadotrophin peak, and second there is good patient acceptability. One disadvantage is possible variability of renal function. This was countered by expressing the gonadotrophin output in relation to urinary creatinine. However, unfortunately, there is little available data on M.O.L.'s for these units. Our own laboratory data would suggest a pre-ovulatory M.O.L. of approximately 7 IU/mmol creatinine and "basal" follicular and luteal levels of circa 3 IU/mmol creatinine.

An additional statistical approach to the gonadotrophin data was to justify the results in terms of the day on which the maximal values occurred. In this situation basal levels are represented on the days occurring 1 day and more remote from the maximal day, and there should be an increase in levels on days adjacent to the maximal day, i.e. a "shoulder" effect, as the gonadotrophin peak occurs over a 2 day interval. The maximal and the "shoulder" levels were compared with the basal levels. In addition in an ovulatory cycle there should be coincidence of the LH and FSH peaks. This was investigated by justifying the FSH data in relation to the LH maximal day, and examining the resulting FSH distribution, and also by a comparison of the actual modal day for maximal levels between the two gonadotrophins.

Results

The peak luteal progesterone levels and all of the follicular phase levels are shown in figure 3. The results have been displayed in this fashion so as to give an immediate visual comparison of all-bold print levels found compared with those expected in the ovulating cycle, and also to show on which days the samples were actually taken. The modal sampling day for the peak luteal level was day 20. It is readily apparent that all of the peak luteal levels were markedly depressed compared with the expected levels of an ovulatory cycle and the levels in fact appear very similar to those found in the follicular phase. The highest luteal phase progesterone level was 1.0 nmol/l.

The results of statistical analysis are shown in table 1. The mean follicular phase level was 0.7 nmol/l and the mean peak luteal value was 0.6 nmol/l. The latter differed significantly from the M.O.L. (15 nmol/l), $P < 0.001$. There was no statistical difference between the peak luteal and mean follicular levels, (paired t test), $P > 0.05$.

The results for the two sub-groups, i.e. those in whom there was a 7 day interval between the two preparations, Group "A", and those in whom there was no such interval, Group "B", are also shown. There was no significant difference ($P > 0.05$) between the mean levels in the two sub-groups.

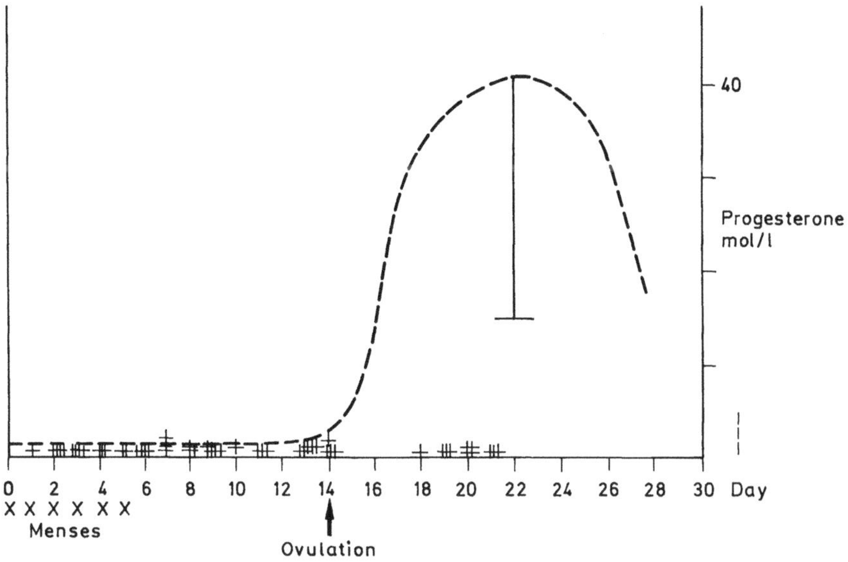

Fig. 3 Progesterone results—peak luteal and total follicular phase

Table 1 Progesterone Results

		Follicular Phase		Peak Luteal Phase	
Total Population					
	Mean	0.7		0.6	
	(SD)	(0.3)		(0.2)	
	nmol/l				
Sub-Populations		A	B	A	B
	Mean	0.6	0.8	0.6	0.7
	(SD)	(0.2)	(0.4)	(0.2)	(0.2)
	nmol/l				

The peak luteal, peak pre-ovulatory and basal levels of estradiol found in the study are shown in figure 4. The modal sampling day for the basal phase was day 2, for the pre-ovulatory peak was day 13, and for the luteal peak day 20. There is no obvious difference between estradiol levels in any of these phases and all of the peak ovulatory and peak luteal results are markedly depressed compared to expected ovulatory cycle levels. The highest pre-ovulatory estradiol level was 199 pmol/l and the highest luteal peak level was 119 pmol/l.

Table 2 shows the results of statistical analysis. The mean basal level was 101 pmol/l, the mean peak pre-ovulatory level was 70 pmol/l, and the mean peak luteal level was 57 pmol/l. Each of the last two differed significantly from

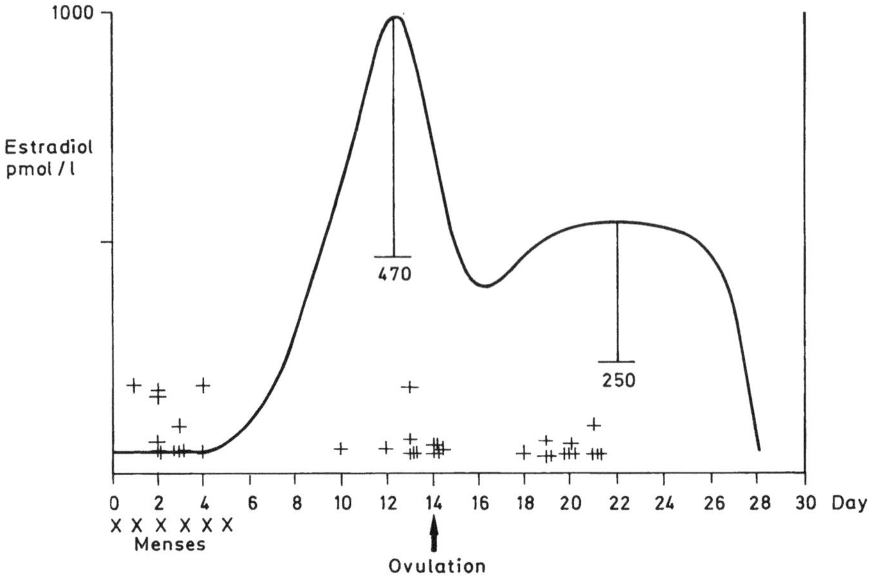

Fig. 4 Estradiol results—peak luteal, peak preovulatory and basal levels

Table 2 Estradiol Results

		Basal		Peak Preovulatory		Peak Luteal	
Total Population							
	Mean	101		70		57	
	(SD)	(65)		(42)		(21)	
	pmol/l						
Sub-Populations		A	B	A	B	A	B
	Mean	106	97	65	73	47	63
	(SD)	(71)	(67)	(14)	(45)	(2)	(25)
	pmol/l						

the respective M.O.L. (470 and 250 pmol/l), $P < 0.001$. In addition there was no statistically significant difference between these three means, (analysis of variance), $P > 0.05$.

The results for the two sub-populations "A" and "B" are also shown. There was no significant difference ($P > 0.05$) between the means at any part of the cycle.

The maximal ovulatory LH levels for each individual are shown in figure 5. The modal sampling day was day 13. These results are obviously depressed compared with the expected ovulatory level of 7 IU/mmol creatinine. The highest recorded level was 3.86 IU/mmol creatinine.

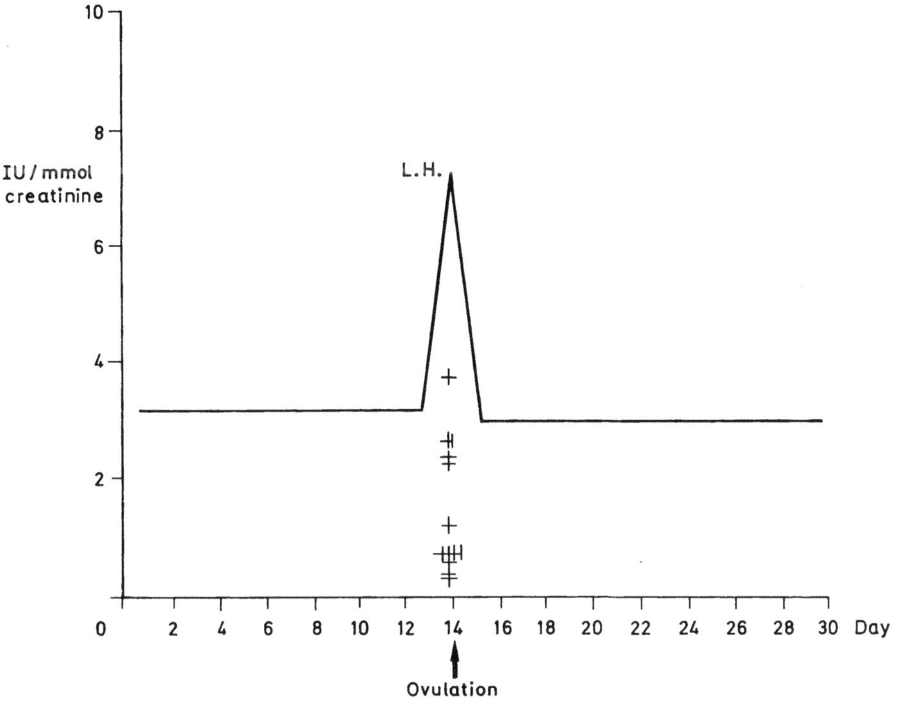

Fig. 5 LH results peak levels (justified to day 14)

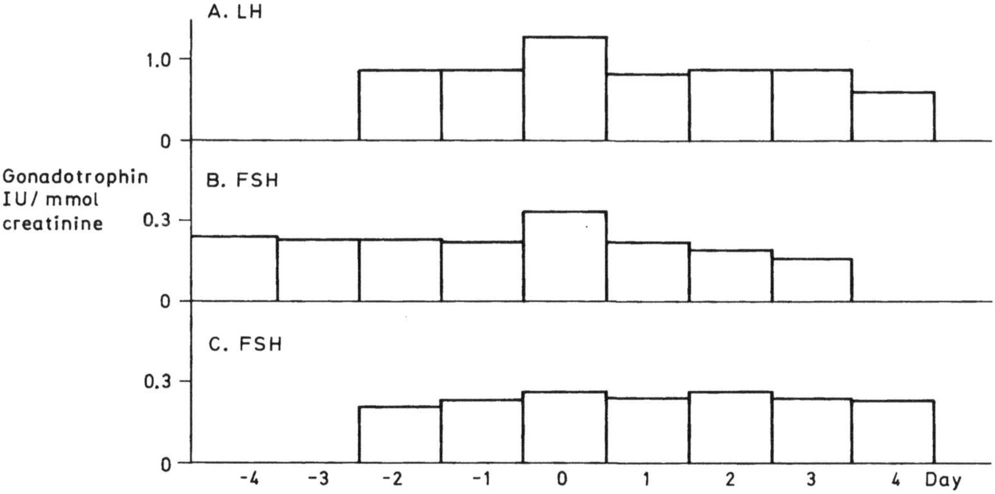

Fig. 6 Gonadotrophin results justified to day of peak level
A. + B.: LH / FSH justified to own day of peak level
C.: FSH justified to LH peak day

Figure 6 A. shows the justified data for LH. There is no obvious "shoulder" effect about the mean. The mean maximal level was 1.3 IU/mmol creatinine and the ratio of this to the mean "basal" level was 1.6, as compared to an expected >2.0 in an ovulatory cycle. Analysis of variance failed to show any statistically significant difference between means of the different days, even including the maximal level. Figure 6 B. shows similar justified data for FSH. Again, there was no obvious "shoulder" effect. The mean maximal FSH level was 0.34 IU/mmol creatinine and the ratio of maximal to "basal" levels was 1.6. No statistically significant difference between means including the maximal levels was found. Fig. 6 C. shows FSH data justified as for the maximal *LH* day. This produced virtual flattening of the FSH distribution, suggesting non-synchronization between LH and FSH excretion. The same result was obtained when the days of occurrence of maximal gonadotrophin levels were compared between LH and FSH with Spearmans Rank Correlation.

Table 3 LH Results

	'Peak' Day		Other Days
Total Population			
Mean	1.28		0.82
(SD)	(0.97)		(0.52)
IU/mmol creatinine			
Sub-Populations	A	B	
Mean	1.57	1.10	
(SD)	(1.36)	(0.67)	
IU/mmol creatinine			

Table 4 FSH Results

	'Peak' Day		Other Days
Total Population			
Mean	0.34		0.21
(SD)	(0.18)		(0.13)
IU/mmol creatinine			
Sub-Populations	A	B	
Mean	0.30	0.37	
(SD)	(0.16)	(0.19)	
IU/mmol creatinine			

Table 3 shows the levels of LH found in the two sub-populations of patients. No significant difference was found between them. Table 4 shows similar results for FSH, and again no significant difference was demonstrated.

Discussion

During the first menstrual cycle of patients taking Diane-35®, following at least three months of Diane-50®, suppression of serum progesterone and estradiol at times of expected peaks has been observed. The data have been analysed by two main approaches, firstly by an external comparison of observed peak levels with minimal expected ovulatory levels (M.O.L.), and secondly by an internal comparison with basal levels. The steroid levels found were profoundly depressed compared with the respective M.O.L.'s, and were also indistinguishable from basal levels of the patients themselves. Therefore, there appeared to be complete suppression of the steroid hormonal cycles, which occurred in all patients.

Gonadotrophin levels were also depressed. The mean maximal ovulatory LH levels were found to be markedly depressed compared to the M.O.L. However, less significance can be given to this, than for the steroid results, as there can be less confidence in the M.O.L. because of the paucity of reference data on ovulatory gonadotrophin levels in small volumes of urine. Accordingly, more emphasis has been placed on internal comparisons. On justification of the data, internal comparisons failed to demonstrate significant differences between maximal and basal levels. Also, there was no evidence of synchronization of maximal values between the two gonadotrophins. These results suggest that there was no true gonadotrophic peak.

There was no detectable difference between patients taking Diane-35® with a 7 day interval following taking Diane-50®, and patients taking Diane-35® on day 1 of the ensuing menstrual loss. It is concluded that ovulation was inhibited in all patients on both dosage regimens.

Summary

A group of 13 patients, who had previously been taking Diane-50® as a treatment for acne for at least three months, were changed to Diane-35®. One subgroup of these patients started the Diane-35® following a 7 day free interval following the Diane-50®, while a second sub-group started the Diane-35® on day 1 of the ensuing menstrual loss.

During the first Diane-35® cycle, there was a complete suppression of the luteal peak progesterone level, pre-ovulatory peak estradiol level and peak luteal estradiol level. There was also no evidence of an ovulatory peak in gonadotrophins, in that maximal levels were both low and desynchronized between LH and FSH.

There was no difference between results in the two dosage regimen subgroups. It is concluded that suppression of ovulation occurred in all patients, irrespective of a dosage regime.

References

[1] Miller, J. A., F. T. Wojnarowska, P. M. Dowd et al.: Antiandrogen treatment in women with acne: A controlled trial. Brit. J. Derm. **114** (1986) 705—716.
[2] Greenwood, R., L. Brummitt, B. Burke et al.: Acne: Double blind clinical and laboratory trial of tetracycline, oestrogen/cyproterone acetate and combined treatment. Brit. Med. J. **291**: (1985) 1231—1235.
[3] Mugglestone, C. J., E. L. Rhodes: The treatment of acne with an antiandrogen/oestrogen combination. Clin. Exp. Derm. **7** (1982) 593—598.
[4] Data on file: Schering Chemicals Ltd. (1985)

Effect of a new antiandrogen-estrogen sub-fifty combination on the endometrium

L. Fedele, M. Marchini, S. G. Carinelli, D. Zamberletti, A. Baglioni

Introduction

Recently a new progestogen-estrogen combination (SHB 209 AE) consisting of cyproterone acetate and low-dose ethinyl estradiol was introduced in clinical studies. It is used in the treatment of some severe manifestations of androgenization, especially when effective contraception is also required.

Clinical results with this preparation have demonstrated a low incidence of intermenstrual spotting and prompt recovery of the cycles after suspension [1].

The aim of the present study was to investigate endometrial modifications induced by SHB 209 AE, using not only light microscopy (LM) but also scanning and transmission electron microscopy (SEM, TEM) in order to demonstrate specific variations of the surface and glandular epithelium.

Materials and methods

We studied 27 volunteers aged between 18 and 35 years who had taken SHB 209 AE during the preceding 3 months. Fifteen of the subjects had acne, seborrhea and hirsutism, 6 had acne and seborrhea, 1 seborrhea and hirsutism, and 5 hirsutism. Contraception was also required by 19.

SHB 209 AE (Diane-35®) is available in tablets each containing 0.035 mg ethinyl estradiol and 2 mg cyproterone acetate that are taken from day 1 of the cycle for 21 consecutive days.

An endometrial biopsy was performed on each patient during the treatment: this was done in the first week in 9 subjects, in the second week in 10 subjects, and in the third week in 8 subjects.

Two or three endometrial fragments with diameter at 2—5 mm were taken from the fundus and posterior wall of the uterus of each patient using a small Novak's curette. Each fragment was subdivided for LM, SEM and TEM examination. The methods of specimen preparation were as previously described [4, 13].

Endometrial biopsies of 15 normally menstruating volunteers taken in the first week of the cycle in six cases, in the second in three, and in the third in six, were used as controls.

The percentage of ciliated compared with non ciliated cells was calculated with Vasquez' method [11] at a magnification of not less than 500 for each biopsy; the number of cilia and microvilli was evaluated by analyzing areas of 5 μ^2.

The counts of ciliated cells, cilia and microvilli were analysed with Student's t-test for paired and non-paired data. $P < 0.05$ was considered significant.

Results

During the first 2 weeks of treatment, the endometrium showed a spectrum of morphological pictures comparable to those of the proliferative phase and of the initial and intermediate secretory phase in most cases [9].

In four cases the endometrium was structurally similar to the proliferative phase (fig. 1) and presented slight superficial edema associated with blood extravasation. The stroma consisted of elongated basophilic cells. The glands, which were tubular and without evident coiling or telescoping (fig. 2), presented irregular secretory features; about 50% of them were lined by acidophilic cells with basal nucleus, and the others by clear cells or by apocrine secretory cells.

In the other cases in which the endometrium simulated the initial or intermediate secretory phase, the stroma consisted of stellate cells with evanescent cytoplasm and occasionally of elongated eosinophilic cells. In some cases slight superficial edema was present with blood extravasation, and in others an initial predecidul transformation and a slight hypertrophy of the spiral arterioles were evident. The glands presented coiling which varied from very slight to appreci-

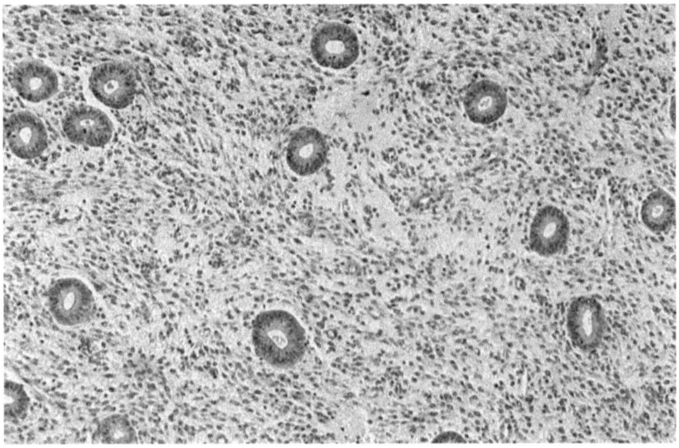

Fig. 1 Endometrium in proliferative phase (control) (H.E. X 40)

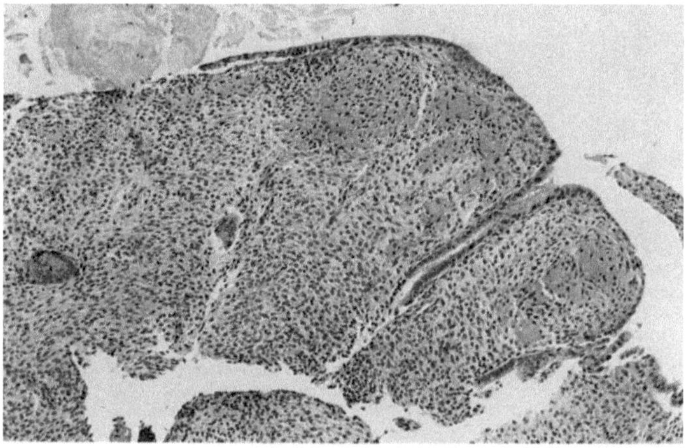

Fig. 2 Week 1st of treatment. Slight superficial edema is evident associated with blood extravasation. The stroma consists of elongated basophilic cells, and the glands present irregular secretory aspects. (H.E. X 10)

able; they were lined by cells of the third-post-ovulatory day type and to a lesser degree by apocrine-type cells.

In only one case was the stroma totally and markedly predecidual with hypertrophic spiral arterioles; the glands presented slight coiling and occasional plugs in the lumen and were lined mainly by eosinophilic-like cells and only sometimes by apocrine-like cells.

At the third week, the surface of all endometria showed focal but marked edema associated with evident micropolypoid hyperplasia (fig. 3). In these regions, in both the superficial stroma and polyps, areas with edematous spindle cells coexisted with other more compact areas. Hyperemia and surface hemor-

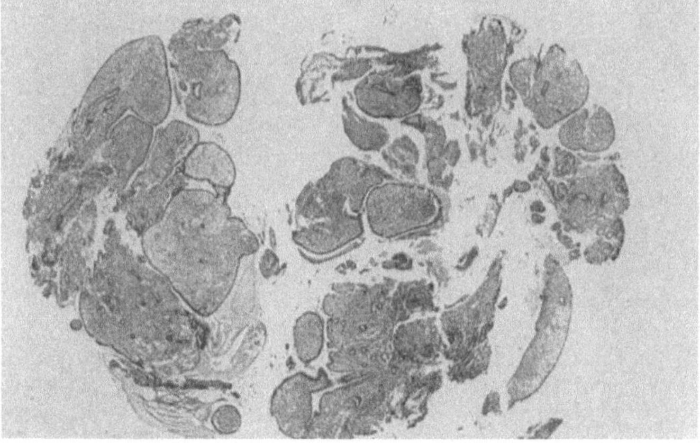

Fig. 3 Week 3rd of treatment. Micropolypoid hyperplasia and foci of superficial edema are observed. (H.E. X 2.5)

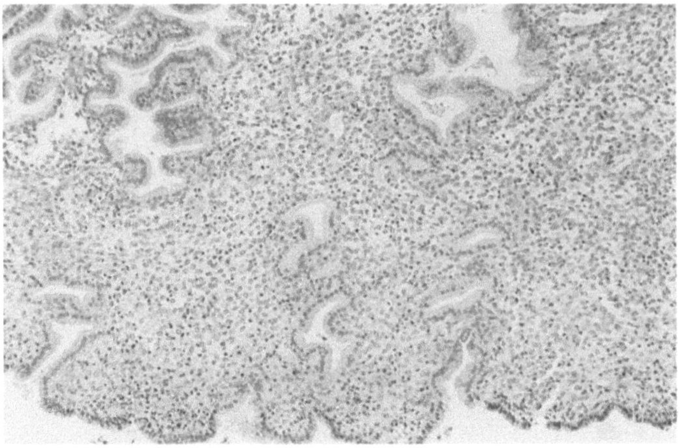

Fig. 4 Endometrium in intermediate secretive phase. (H.E. X 10)

rhages were observed in the former area. These were particularly evident in two cases of completly predecidual endometrium.

Glandular coiling was practically absent, whereas telescoping, although slight, was present. The type of glands was relatively homogeneous due to the absolute prevalence of apocrine-secretory like and eosinophilic cells. Glands lined by clear cells were observed in only two cases. The diameter of the glands varied; however, it was always less than that found in the control endometria (fig. 4).

The greatest degree of gland dilatation was observed in the first and second weeks. Cases in which the glands were extremely restricted were seen only in the first and third weeks.

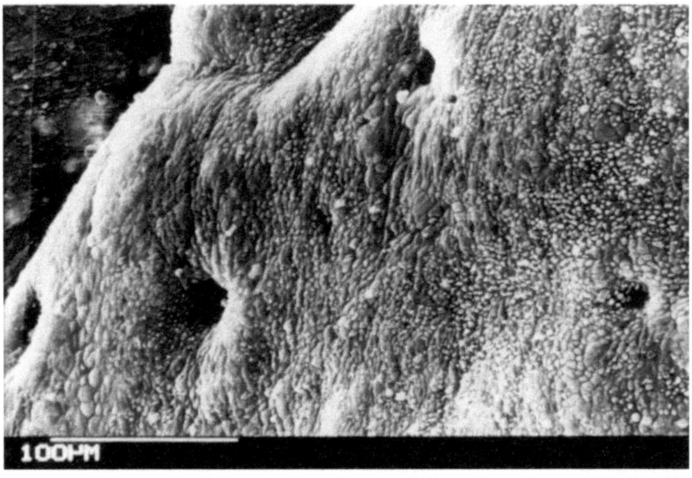

Fig. 5 Aspects of control endometrium in proliferative phase. (SEM X 200)

Mitosis was observed occasionally in the glands of 14 of the 27 cases and in the stroma in 24 of the 27 during all three weeks of treatment.

After 3 days of treatment, it was already possible to distinguish the ciliated cells and non-ciliated cells at SEM. Their ratio in the controls was 1 : 100 (fig. 5); in the treated patients it was 1 : 130, and in some cases 1 : 150. The ratio was almost the same at the end of the first week of treatment.

The distribution of ciliated cells and gland lumina on the endometrial surface was irregular. Areas completely lacking in cilia (delayed ciliogenesis) could be demonstrated (fig. 6).

Compared with the controls, the non-ciliated cells had much blunter and rarer microvilli (52 ± 16 per 5 μ^2 versus 67 ± 19 per 5 μ^2, $P < 0.01$). On days 5—6 the loss of homogeneity of the endometrial surface typical of progestogen-estrogen treatment was evident.

After 13—14 days of treatment the distribution of the gland lumina on the endometrial surface remained more irregular than in the controls, and without significant change in density in relation to the first week of treatment. Initial elongation of the gland lumina was present less frequently than in the control endometria.

At this time the ciliated cells were more numerous than during the proliferative phase (the ciliated/non-ciliated cell ratio was 1: 65 halfway through the cycle, 1: 130 during the first week of treatment), but always notably lower than in the controls (1: 120). The cellular density of the cilia was significantly lower than in the controls (61 ± 12 per 5 μ^2 versus 70 ± 15 per 5 μ^2, $P < 0.05$), but higher than during the early proliferative phase.

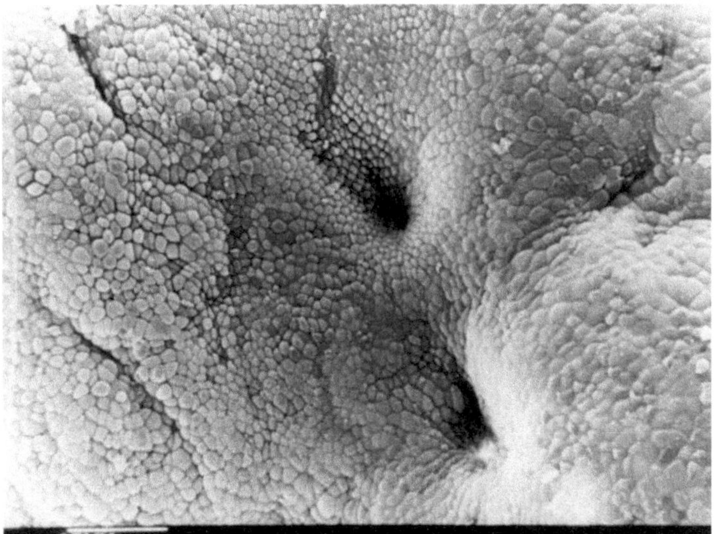

Fig. 6 End of week 1st of treatment. Irregular distribution of the scanty ciliated cells. (SEM X 500)

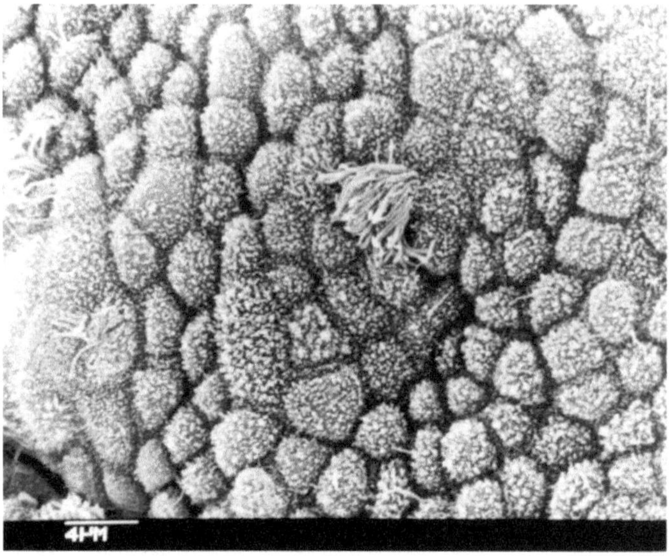

Fig. 7 Week 2nd of treatment. The nonciliated cells present rare and irregularly distributed microvilli. (SEM X 5000)

In the patients in the treatment group the number of microvilli was higher than in the preceding phase (65 ± 18 per 5 μ^2 versus 52 ± 15 per 5 μ^2, $P<0.01$), but lower than in the controls (79 ± 11 per 5 μ^2, $P<0.01$) (fig. 7).

Halfway through the secretory phase (at 20—22 days of treatment) the endometrial surface showed the characteristics of irregularity and maturity typical of progestogen-estrogen treatment; the distribution of the gland lumina was more irregular than that of the controls, and the form of the gland ostia was rarely ellipsoidal as in normal epithelium.

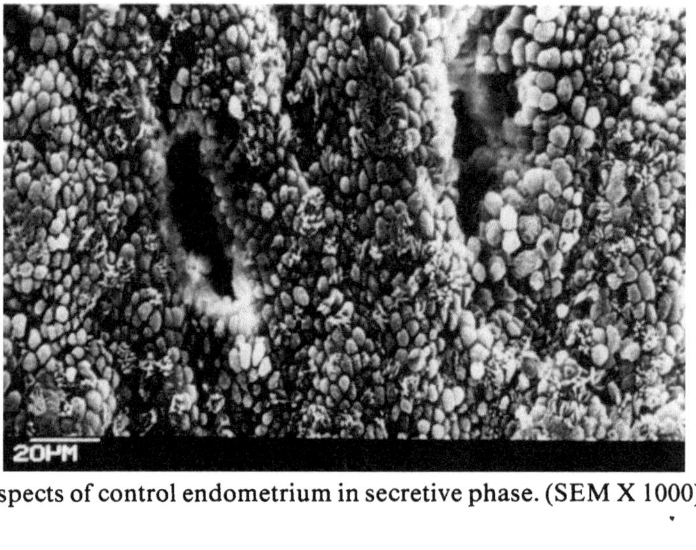

Fig. 8 Aspects of control endometrium in secretive phase. (SEM X 1000)

The ciliated/non-ciliated cells ratio (1 : 59) did not vary significantly with respect to the cycle halfway point although it was still markedly lower than in the controls. Ciliary density was slightly but not significantly, lower than in the preceding phase (55 ± 6 per 5 μ^2 versus 59 ± 7 per 5 μ^2, $P < 0.05$) and notably lower than in the controls (67 ± 21 per 5 μ^2, $P < 0.01$).

The non-ciliated cells showed only a minimal degree of the typically swollen and dome-shaped characteristics that, in the normal endometrium, indicates increased cellular secretory activity.

In the endometria of the treated patients an inhibition of growth of the microvilli was observed. These were blunter and rarer than in the controls (72 ± 19 per 5 μ^2 versus 93 ± 21 per 5 μ^2, $P < 0.05$) but not significantly changed compared with the preceding phase (65 ± 12 per 5 μ^2).

Apocrine secretion in the endometria of the treated patients was, on the average, less than in the controls (fig. 8). However, initial secretion appeared earlier: on the 16—17 day of treatment.

Ultrastructural observation of the various organelles at TEM showed notable differences to those of the control endometria. In the first week fewer mitochondria with rare and only slightly electron-dense cristae could be observed in cells of the glandular epithelium than in the controls. Also the RER, although as abundant as in the control endometria, consisted of irregular, serpiginous cisternae packed together towards the cytoplasmic membrane. Glycogen deposits were scarcely detectable, whereas the number of lipid droplets was comparable to that in the control endometria.

All the epithelial cells were separated by a wide intercellular space occupied by numerous cytoplasmic projections; this was rarely the case in the controls.

Stromal cellularity was scanty; cells had long cytoplasmic projections connected by gap junctions. There were fewer cytoplasmic organelles than in the controls, especially fewer Golgi apparati and lipid droplets. In this phase, the moderate mitotic activity which could be observed in the control endometria seemed to be absent in the endometria of the patients treated with SHB 209 AE.

At days 10—12 some changes were observed: the glandular cells that had been arranged in a monolining were now multilayered, and, compared with the preceding week, a moderate increase could be seen in the number and size of the microvilli. These latter were still, however, blunter and rarer than in the controls, and were often intertwined.

Early secretory characteristics were also evident in the epithelial cells: their apexes were occupied by numerous vacuoles; sometimes there was also a more electron-dense pole, and glycogen deposits. In this phase the number of Golgi apparati was higher than in the preceding weeks. As in the controls, the mitochondria retained the same features as presented in the first days of the cycle although, halfway through the cycle they were often surrounded by cisternae of RER that decreased as treatment continued.

Stromal cellularity was greater than in the previous observation, but less than in the controls, thus presenting precocious edematous aspects typical of pre-decidualization.

At days 18—20 the secretory features which were seen halfway through the cycle had not developed completely; although the number of vacuoles and of mono and pluriparticulate glycogen deposits increased as it did in the controls, signs of apocrine secretion such as the apical cell membrane rupture, which were typical in the control endometria were not visible.

Also the microvilli did not undergo further development. Ciliated cells were observed only in this phase. Those, however, had a markedly reduced and inadequate number of cilia compared with the controls.

The nucleus of the epithelial cells, which was located centrally, slowly shifted towards the basal pole of the cell.

The stromal cells were more roundish, scattered in abundant intercellular substance, and richer in organelles than during the preceding weeks. They did not, however, achieve the development of the control endometria.

Discussion

The endometria of patients on SHB 209 AE treatment presented a shortened proliferative phase in which growth of the structures was reduced compared with that of the normal cycle. In the first 2 weeks of treatment, patterns were observed which were comparable to a proliferative phase and to an initial secretory phase. These had no clear relation to the duration of treatment. Furthermore, the glands did not present the degree of coiling and dilatation found in the normal menstrual cycle [2, 3].

On the other hand, during the entire duration of the treatment mitosis was observed in both the glands and stroma, demonstrating constant proliferation.

Another characteristic was secretory activity of the glands during the entire treatment period. In the first 2 weeks features typical of the third postovulatory day were frequent, whereas during the third week secretory features similar to the advanced secretory phase prevailed (secretion in the lumen and emptying of the apocrine cells). However, even in the most "proliferative" endometria, there was no lack of glands lined by apocrine secretory cells or by clear cells.

The stroma underwent an early predecidual transformation, which was probably preceded by a phase of edema. As with other types of progestogen-estrogen combination, there was a micropolypoid transformation of the endometrium. However, a decidual transformation did not take place [7, 10].

Although surface edema was frequently present during the entire treatment period, there was a lower incidence of intermenstrual spotting reported by the patients. This may be explained by the absence of dilated capillaries.

Under the SEM, with low magnification, a typical loss of homogeneity of the endometrial surface which was characterized by modifications affecting the various endometrial components could be seen. The ciliated cells were significantly less numerous than in the control endometria in all phases of the cycle. As in the controls, their number and ratio with nonciliated cells was greatest halfway through the cycle [8]. However, ciliogenesis was always notably delayed compared with the normal endometrium during the various cycle phases. Also development of the cilia was also notably altered, with the cilia usually reduced in number, shorter, and blunter than in the controls.

Under the TEM it could be seen that the ultrastructure of the cilia retained the normal constitution of nine peripheral filaments and two central filaments.

The nonciliated cells increased during the secretory phase, as in the control endometria, but showed only to a minimal degree the typical swollen and dome-shaped appearance that, in the normal endometrium, demonstrates increased cellular secretory activity. These findings were confirmed by the ultrastructural images obtained by the TEM: These showed fewer mitochondria with slightly rarer cristae than in the controls and RER suggesting a generic decrease in cell activity. The intracellular deposits of mono and pluriparticulate glycogen were scanty.

The microvillous field, which in the control endometria reached maximum development on days 23—25 of the cycle, was always notably reduced in the endometria of the patients on treatment, indicating that growth of the microvilli was inhibited. Also, the ultrastructure of the microvilli differed from those in the controls in that they were were shorter, blunter and not as regularly distributed on the cell surface.

Although the appearance of signs of apocrine secretion in the endometria of the treated patients occurred, on the average, earlier than in the controls, but it was decreased overall. The ultrastructural study showed, however, that the proliferative phase of the cycle was shortened; the cellular components, their differentation (cilia and microvilli) and the gland openings did not ever develop completely.

Similarly, secretory modifications (early apocrine secretion and elongation of the gland lumina seen under the SEM as well as accumulation of glycogen deposits in the apical portion of the cell seen under the TEM) appeared prematurely and remained incomplete. The above-described ultrastructural aspects of the surface were maintained without important alterations even in the secretory phase. There was then a clear contrast between the image of the normal endometrium and that on progestogen-estrogen treatment which presented as irregular, scarcely trophic and with frankly hyposecretory aspects.

Compared with the endometrium on treatment with other progestogen-estrogen combinations, the surface of the endometria on SHB 209 AE treatment demonstrated fewer gland openings. A monomorphic endometrial surface was observed, as described by other authors [5, 6, 12]. This mainly consisted of non-ciliated cells with blunt microvilli, mostly conglutinated, and with scanty secretory material.

The nucleus of the glandular cells, which was located in the intermediate cell segment in the first week, migrated towards the basal pole of the cell in the two subsequent weeks. The presence of an increased number of vacuoles, glycogen deposits, and moderatly well developed Golgi cisternae in the apical portion of the glandular cells was not, however, comparable to that in the control endometria, in which the frank secretory activity was shown by rupture of the cytoplasmic membrane and the consequent release of the content into the gland lumen.

Conclusion

Our histomorphologic investigation demonstrated an overall weak growth of the endometrial mucosa which presented early, but weak, secretory modifications and which did not develop completely.

The stroma also showed early predecidual aspects, sometimes accompanied by slight hypertrophy of the spiral arterioles.

Capillary dilatation was markedly decreased, which may explain the rare intermenstrual spotting and/or tardy secretory phase.

The most characteristic modifications of the surface epithelium of the human endometrium on treatment with SHB 209 AE were:

- A reduction of the ciliated cells compared with the nonciliated cells. This reduction was constant during all 3 weeks of treatment, although at the end of the second week it tended to become less marked.
- Insufficient secretory modifications which cause the apocrine phenomena, appeared in the first week, but remained incomplete during the entire treatment. These modifications caused a total alteration of the mucosal architecture and cellular maturation that compromised the implantation phase.

The ultrastructure seen under the TEM demonstrated a reduced activity of the epithelial cells that manifested in scanty development of the cytoplasmic organelles (mitochondria and RER). Secretory activity was documented by the accumulation of mono and pluriparticulate glycogen; however, apocrine maturation was reduced, making the secretory activity insufficient.

References

[1] Cavalli, G., L. Fedele, D. Zamberletti et al.: Clinical effects of a new monophasic oral contraceptive with antiandrogenic activity (SHB 209 AE) in 458 treatment cycles. Program and abstracts of First International Congress on Gynecological Endocrinology. March 16—22, 1986 Madonna di Campiglio.

[2] Dallenbach-Hellweg, D.: Histopathology of the Endometrium. pp. 24—38. Springer-Verlag, New York 1971.
[3] Demopulos, R. I.: Normal endometrium. In: Blaustein (Ed.): Pathology of the female tract. Second edition, pp. 234—278. Springer-Verlag, New York 1982.
[4] Fedele, L., G. Cavalli, M. Marchini: Effect of a new oral antiandrogen-estrogen combination on the endometrium: histological and ultrastructural scanning electron microscopy study. Acta Eur. Fertil. **17** (1986) 9—13.
[5] Ferenczy, A.: Surface ultrastructural reponse of the human uterine lining epithelium to hormonal environment a scanning electron microscopy study. Acta Cytol. **21** (1977) 566—572.
[6] Ferenczy, A., R. M. Richart: Scanning and transmission electron microscopy of the human endometrial surface epithelium. J. Clin. Endocrin. Metabol. **36** (1973) 999—1008.
[7] Goldzieher, J. W., M. Maqueo et al.: Comparative studies of the ethinyl estrogens used in oral contraceptives. Am. J. Obstet. Gynecol. **122** (1975) 615—618.
[8] Ludwig, H., H. Metzeger: The human female reproductive tract. A scanning electron microscopic atlas, pp. 31—78. Springer-Verlag, New York 1976.
[9] Noyes, R. H., A. T. Hertig, J. Rock: Dating the endometrial biopsy. Fertil. Steril. **1** (1950) 3.
[10] Song, J., M. S. Mark, M. P. Lawler: Endometrial changes in women receiving oral contraceptives. Am. J. Obstet. Gynecol. **107** (1970) 717—728.
[11] Vasquez, G., R. M. L. Winston: The epithelium of human hydrosalpinges a light and scanning electron microscopy study. Br. J. Ob. Gynec. **90** (1983) 764.
[12] Wienke, E. C., F. Cavazos, D. G. Hall: Ultrastructural effects of norethynodrel and mestranol on human endometrial stroma cell. Am. J. Obstet. Gynecol. **103** (1969) 102—111.
[13] Zamberletti, D., R. Rainoldi, M. Sideri: Significato delle modificazioni dell'epitelio di superficie dell'endometrio nel corso del ciclo mestruale. Ann. Ost. Gin. Med. Perin. **103** (1982) 113—119.

II Polycystic ovary syndrome

Endocrinological and clinical findings on the therapy with Diane-35® in polycystic ovary syndrome

L. Falsetti, G. A. Casarotti, A. Gastaldi

Introduction

The polycystic ovary syndrome (PCOS) is certainly the most frequently occurring endocrine pathology in women in fertile age: its incidence varies from 1.5% to 3.5% [1].

Estrogen-progestins (E/P) are widely used for the long term therapy of the polycystic ovary syndrome. The use of these drugs is justified by their mechanism of action: during treatment reduced LH excretion and a decrease in the amount of ovarian androgens are obtained [2, 3]. Moreover, estrogen-progestins were shown to inhibit adrenal androgen production (dehydroepiandrosterone and dehydroepiandrosterone sulphate). The mechanism by which adrenal suppression takes place is not yet entirely understood. Carr et al. have observed that in normal women the intake of oral contraceptives results in a decrease of ACTH plasma levels [5]. The effect of estrogen-progestins on ACTH could be mediated by the variations of transcortin, of cortisol and of its metabolic clearance rate (MCR). In fact the decrease of dehydroepiandrosterone sulphate (DHEA-S) plasma concentrations seems to be correlated with the plasma ACTH decrease. Moreover, it has been proved that estrogen-progestins inhibit delta-5-pregnenolone synthesis [7]. It must also be considered that DHEA-S reduction may be attributed to the suppression that estrogen-progestins exert on the ovarian steroidogenesis and thus even on DHEA quota. Lobo et al. showed a significant relationship between bio-LH and DHEA-S in patients with PCOS, suggesting that biologically active LH may exert a direct influence on the adrenal gland [8]. A further characteristic of estrogen-progestins is that they induce an increase in the binding globulin (SHBG) produced by the liver, and a subsequent decrease in free androgens in the blood [3—9]. Such a biological mechanism supported by estradiol (E_2) also partly depends on both the type of progestin used and its degree of androgenicity. Cyproterone acetate (CPA), a progestin derivate of 17-α-hydroxy-progesterone, supresses adrenal gland activity (demonstrated in animals but not yet completely in man), and has a marked antigonadotropic action as well as a peripheric antiandrogen action (competition for androgen receptor and inhibition of receptor binding) [10, 12, 12]. In our study we used the new association ethinyl estradiol 0.035 mg/cyproterone acetate 2 mg (Diane-35®) in patients with PCOS throughout the 2 years [11, 12].

In contrast to other studies reported in literature where the combination of 0.05 mg ethinyl estradiol and 2 mg cyproterone acetate was used in groups of nonhomogeneous patients for the treatment at the basic endocrine pathology, our study used a low-dosage ethinyl estradiol/cyproterone acetate combination for PCOS therapy.

Materials and methods

We selected 24 women with PCOS, among them 23 with clinical hyperandrogenic symptoms (acne, seborrhea, hirsutism), with ages ranging from 16 to 32 years (mean age: 23.5 ± 4.7 years), from a group of patients that came to the Centre of Gynecologic Endocrinology in the Departments of Obstetrics and Gynecology, University of Brescia (Italy). The diagnosis of PCOS was made according to the characteristic endocrine (tab. 1) and clinical patterns: constantly high LH (30.8 ± 6.2 mIU/ml) with a LH/FSH ratio of 3.01 and androgens with higher than normal plasma concentrations (androstenedione (A) 3.4 ± 0.8 ng/ml, total testosterone (T.Te) 0.9 ± 0.2 ng/ml, free testosterone (F.Te) 19.2 + 2.1 pg/ml, DHEA-S = 4.0 ± 0.9 μg/ml). Hormone values were obtained from an average of 3 determinations.

The clinical picture is shown in table 2. The body mass index (BMI) was 22.2 and 8 women were overweight (33.3%). Ten presented secondary amenorrhea (41.7%) and 10 oligomenorrhea (41.7%).

Androgenic symptoms were the following: acne in 21 women (87.5%), seborrhea in 23 (95.8%) and hirsutism in 18 (75%). No patient wanted children or had

Table 1 BASAL ENDOCRINE PARAMETERS

LH	mUI/ml	30.8 ± 6.2
FSH	mUI/ml	10.2 ± 2.0
PRL	ng/ml	11.5 ± 4.4
E_1	pg/ml	90.5 ± 14.9
E_2	pg/ml	62.2 ± 13.4
A	ng/ml	3.4 ± 0.8
T.TE	ng/ml	0.9 ± 0.3
F.TE	pg/ml	19.2 ± 2.1
DHEA-S	ug/ml	4.0 ± 0.9
LH/FSH	ratio	3.01
E_1/E_2	ratio	1.44
SHBG	nMol/1	35.4 ± 10.4

Table 2 BASAL CLINICAL PARAMETERS

Mean age of menarche	13.2				
Body mass index (BMI)*	22.2				
Overweight patients	8	(33.3%)			
Oligomenorrhea	10	(41.7%)			
Amenorrhea II	10	(41.7%)			
Regular cycles	4	(16.6%)			
Acne	21	(87.5%)	Moderate	15	(71.4%)
			Severe	6	(28.6%)
Seborrhea	23	(95.8%)	Moderate	11	(47.8%)
			Severe	12	(52.2%)
Hirsutism	18	(75.0%)	Mild	5	(27.8%)
			Moderate	8	(44.4%)
			Severe	5	(27.8%)

* Body mass index
Acceptable: 18–23.5; over weight: 23.5–29.5; obese: 29.5–38

any contraindication to the use of oral contraceptives. We suggested that each of the 24 patients started taking the monophasic "pill" (Diane-35®) containing ethinyl estradiol 0.035 mg and cyproterone acetate 2 mg for a period of 2 years.

Each woman was given a calendar and instructed how to record the days on which the pill was taken and the secondary effects observed. The study program included endocrine and clinical check-ups. The endocrine follow-up performed at the 6th, 12th, and 24th treatment cycle included the assessment of LH, FSH, prolactin (PRL), estrone (E_1), 17β estradiol (E_2), A, T.Te, F.Te, DHEA-S. Moreover, the behaviour of sex hormone binding globulin (SHBG) was investigated and found to show basic values of 35.4 ± 10.3 nMol/l in our group of patients with PCOS (normal values in the follicular phase of the cycle: 66 ± 26.7 nMol/l).

Hormonal dosage was performed by RIA technique with commercial kits from Biodata, Serono, and Sorin; SHBG by the IRMA method of Farmos. In particular, F.Te was determined by a RIA method developed at the Institute of Chemistry, University of Brescia (Italy) (normal values for the women of fertile age and in follicular phase: 6.03 ± 2.9 pg/ml).

Clinical follow-ups were performed at the 6th, 12th, 18th and 24th treatment cycles. The physical examination schedule included the following check-ups: for "acne", face, neck base, back; for "seborrhea", skin, hair, dandruff; for "hirsutism", face, chest, abdomen and lower limbs. In order to obtain a rating of symptoms and therapeutic results, the findings relating to each body area were converted to an overall evaluation of the symptom itself according to a score. In this way seborrhea and acne could be subdivided into moderate and severe forms.

Every three months, all women underwent a follow-up consisting of a check of body weight and arterial blood pressure and a reading of the calendar-form. They were also questioned about the onset of side effects. Of the 24 patients, 4 stopped taking the drug after 12 cycles and 1 after 18, not because of side effects or intolerance towards the pill, but for personal reasons.

Results

The outcome of our study can be broken down into endocrine and clinical findings.

a) Endocrine findings

Table 3 shows the changes of all the hormones we took into consideration and of the SHBG during the 24 treatment cycles. The significant suppression of all hormones except PRL and the surprising increase of SHBG during treatment with this drug are evident. Moreover, there is a further marked decrease of E_2 and A from the 6th to the 12th treatment cycle. At the endocrine check-up after 24 treatment cycles, the hormone picture is the same as the one after 12 treatment cycles except that F.Te values show a further significant decrease. Gonadotropin (GN) blood levels drop to perfectly normal values (LH = 8.5 ± 7.8 – FSH = 5.6 ± 3.8 mUI/ml) after only 6 treatment cycles. At the 12th treatment cycle follow-up examination a further decrease of LH (5.7 ± 3.2 mUI/ml) and FSH (5.3 ± 3.9 mUI/ml) can be noticed. These remain almost unchanged at the 24th treatment cycle. The LH/FSH ratio decreases considerably at the 6th cycle (3.01 → 1.51) with a further drop that settles to steady values at the 12th and 24th treatment cycles (1.07 → 1.18). The estrogen decrease is already signi-

Table 3 ENDCOCRINE PARAMETERS

		BASAL	6th CYCLE	12th CYCLE	24th CYCLE
LH	mUI/ml	30.8 ± 6.2°	8.5 ± 7.8°	5.7 ± 3.2	5.8 ± 3.2
FSH	mUI/ml	10.2 ± 2.0°	5.6 ± 3.8°	5.3 ± 3.9	4.9 ± 1.9
PRL	ng/ml	11.5 ± 4.4	11.6 ± 4.9	10.6 ± 3.7	9.6 ± 3.7
E_1	pg/ml	90.5 ± 14.9°	30.8 ± 13.9°	29.6 ± 11.6	27.2 ± 8.5
E_2	pg/ml	62.2 ± 13.4°	46.7 ± 18.4°*	23.2 ± 10.3*	23.9 ± 9.7
A	ng/ml	3.4 ± 0.8°	1.8 ± 0.7°*	1.3 ± 0.5*	1.3 ± 0.5
T.Te	ng/ml	0.9 ± 0.3°	0.5 ± 0.3°	0.5 ± 0.2	0.5 ± 0.2
F.Te	pg/ml	19.2 ± 2.1°	7.1 ± 2.2°	8.6 ± 3.3▪	6.6 ± 1.8▪
DHEA-S	μg/ml	4.0 ± 0.9°	2.1 ± 1.2°	2.0 ± 0.7	1.7 ± 0.4
LH/FSH	ratio	3.01	1.51	1.07	1.18
E_1/E_2	ratio	1.44	0.09	1.17	1.13
SHBG	nMol/1	35.4 ± 10.4°	206.3 ± 52°	193.6 ± 63.9	188.0 ± 39.2

° $P < 0.01$ * $P < 0.01$ ▪ $P < 0.05$

ficant at the 6th treatment cycle follow-up examination (E_1 = 30.8 ± 13.9 pg/ml). Moreover, E_2 shows a further decrease at the 12th cycle (E_2 = 23.2 ± 10.3 pg/ml). During the last year of treatment E_1 and E_2 values did not vary.

Androgens decrease progressively until the 12th treatment cycle; they pass from basic values of 3.4 ± 0.8 ng/ml to 1.3 ± 0.5 ng/ml and remain unchanged at the examination carried out at the end of the trial. T.Te, after the drop of the values found at the 6th cycle (0.5 ± 0.3 ng/ml), is not changed at the 12th and 24th cycle (0.5 ± 0.2 ng/ml). On the other hand, F.Te shows a progressive decrease: in fact, after a highly significant decrease ($P < 0.01$) at the 6th cycle (19.2 ± 2.1 → 7.1 ± 2.3 pg/ml), it shows a stabilisation of values between the 6th and 12th cycle and then decreases significantly ($P < 0.05$) at the 24th cycle of treatment (6.6 ± 1.8 pg/ml).

DHEA-S shows a maximal decrease at the 6th treatment cycle (4.0 ± 0.9 → 2.1 ± 1.2 µg/ml) and settles to steady values which are maintained until the end of the trial.

As far as SHBG are concerned, this new ethinyl estradiol/cyproterone acetate combination is able to increase more than 5 times the values found in basic conditions (basic = 35.4 ± 10 → 24 cycles = 188 + 39.2 nMol/l).

b) Clinical findings

The changes in hyperandrogenic symptoms (acne, seborrhea, hirsutism) observed during the treatment with this drug are shown in tables 4, 5, and 6 and in figures 1, 2, and 3.

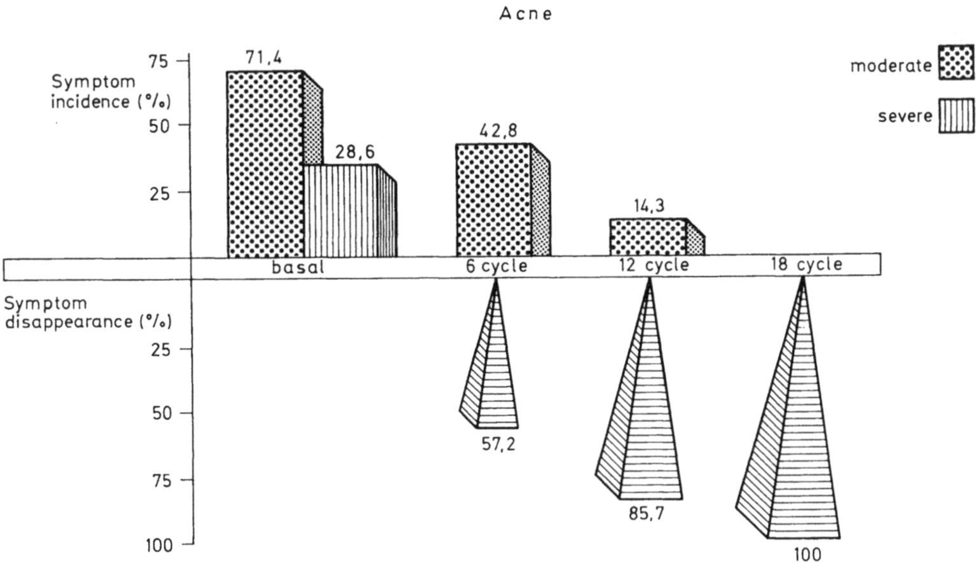

Fig. 1 Changes in acne during treatment with Diane-35®

Table 4 ACNE

	BASAL	6th CYCLE	12th CYCLE	18th CYCLE	24th CYCLE
N. cases	21	21	21	19	18
Moderate	15 (71.4%)	9 (42.8%)	3 (14.3%)	0	0
Severe	6 (28.6%)	0	0	0	0
Disappearance of sympton (%)	–	57.2	85.7	100	100
Recovered pts.	–	12	18	19	18

Acne (tab. 4, fig. 1) was present in 21 (87.5%) women before treatment: 15 (71.4%) moderate and 6 (28.6%) severe. Analysis of the changes during the 2 years of treatment, showed that acne reduces progressively, disappearing in all patients between the 12th and 18th treatment cycle. At the 6th treatment cycle follow-up examination 12 (57%) patients were found to be completely cured and the remaining 9 patients were partly cured—they showed only a moderate form. Seborrhea (tab. 5, fig. 2) was present in 23 (95.8%) women: 11 (47.8%) moderate and 12 (52.2%) severe. The treatment turned out to be very effective for this symptom: at the 12th cycle a complete recovery of 52.2% of patients and disappearance of the severe forms was observed. After that the results did not vary significantly.

Hirsutism (tab. 6, fig. 3) was present at the beginning in 18 (75%) women: 27.8% mild, 44.4% moderate and 27.8% severe. A global analysis of the symptom in its evolution, showed that already at the 6th treatment cycle it has disappeared completely in 4 (22.2%) women and partly in the others. The severe form no longer occurs. A further progressive improvement can be noticed leading to a complete absence of moderate forms at the 24th cycle. Mild hirsutism is then present only in 33.3% of the patients (n = 5).

Of the 4 symptomatic women lost during the trial, 3 left after having completed the 12th cycle and 1 at the 18th cycle. On entrance to the trial, seborrhea was present in 4 patients (1 severe form, 3 moderate forms), hirsutism in 3 cases (1 severe form, 1 moderate form, 1 mild form), acne in 3 (all moderate forms). At voluntary interruption of therapy, 2 patients showed hirsutism in a mild form; all the other symptoms had clinically disappeared.

Table 5 SEBORRHEA

	BASAL	6th CYCLE	12th CYCLE	18th CYCLE	24th CYCLE
N. cases	23	23	23	20	19
Moderate	11 (47.8%)	12 (52.2%)	11 (47,8%)	8 (40.0%)	8 (42.0%)
Severe	12 (52.2%)	3 (13.1%)	0	0	0
Disappearance of symptom (%)	–	34.7	52.2	60	58
Recovered pts.	–	8	12	12	11

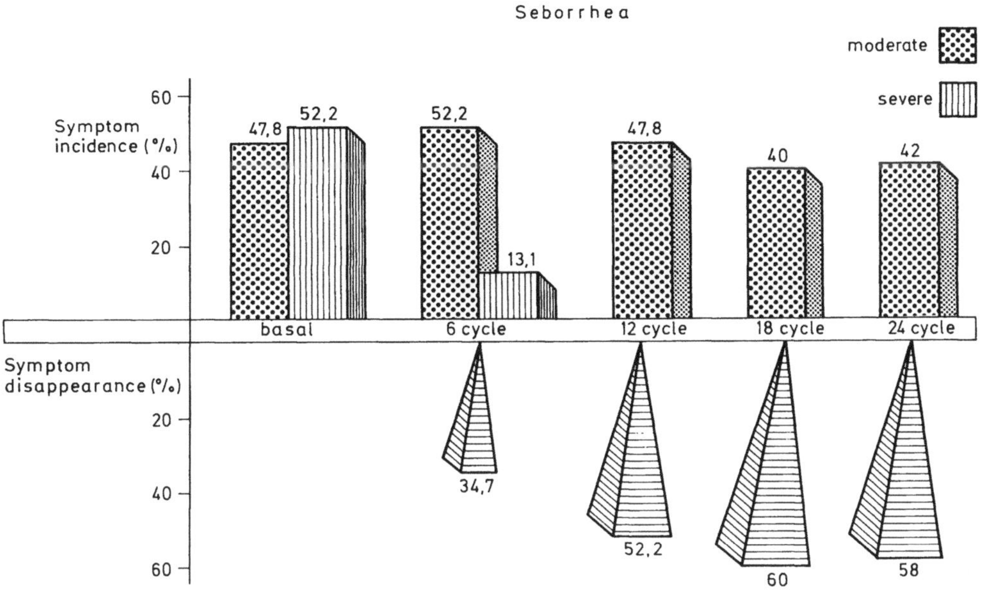

Fig. 2 Changes in seborrhea during treatment with Diane-35®

Summing up, we can conclude that the rate of disappearance for each symptom of hyperandrogenism is as follows: acne 100% at the 18th cycle (fig. 1), seborrhea 52% and 58% at the 12th and 24th cycles (fig. 2), respectively, and hirsutism 66.7% at the 24th cycle (fig. 3). The cycle was always kept under control during the entire 24 cycles treatment period and no pregnancy occurred. Body weight and arterial blood pressure did not show any significant change.

Table 6 HIRSUTISM

	BASAL	6th CYCLE	12th CYCLE	18th CYCLE	24th CYCLE
N. cases	18	18	18	15	15
Mild	5 (27.8%)	5 (27.8%)	7 (38,9%)	4 (26.7%)	5 (33.3%)
Moderate	8 (44.0%)	9 (50.0%)	3 (16,7%)	3 (20.0%)	0
Severe	5 (27.8%)	0	0	0	0
Disappearance of symptom (%)	–	22.2	44.4	53.3	66.7
Recovered pts.	–	4	8	8	10

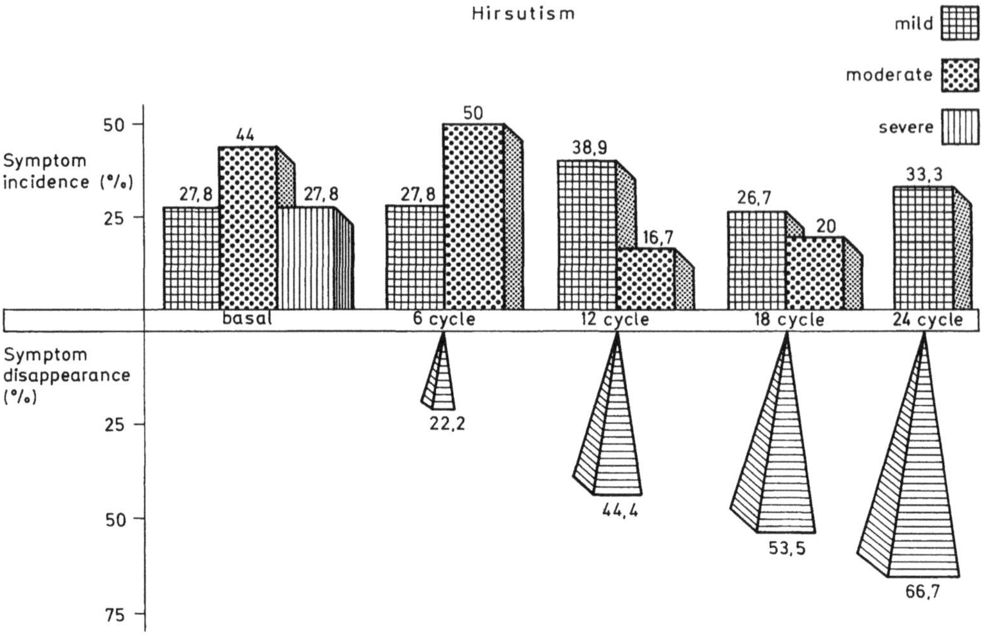

Fig. 3 Changes in hisutism during treatment with Diane-35®

Discussion

Estrogen-progestins have been employed in the therapy of PCOS to correct the endocrine profile and improve hyperandrogenism symptoms for a long time. The use of the pill must, however, be limited to women of less than forty years of age who do not want children and who show no contraindication to the use of oral contraceptives. Moreover, a choice has to be made as to the hormone dosage, the molecular structure of the progestins and the need for a long term therapy. The following estrogen-progestins have to be ruled out "a priori": sequential pill, pills with progestins derived from 19-nortestosterone. Furthermore, pills with high-dosage estrogens cannot be used because of the greater risk of cardiovascular complications. In our view, the pill with the lowest dose of estrogen that at the same time is effective in modifying the endocrine profile, above all the LH values, should be used. Considering all these factors, we carried out this study to, above all, verify whether an estrogen-progestin combination containing 0.035 mg of ethinyl estradiol could change the endocrine parameters of PCOS and, therefore, present a therapeutic strategy. From the data in the literature, the conclusion can be drawn that the therapeutical effectiveness of estrogen-progestins for PCOS is tied to two fundamental factors: an appropriate steroid dosage and estrogenic hormonal profile. In fact many authors maintain that in order to obtain an inhibition of the release of LH, the pill must contain not only an appropriate dose of progestins, but also more than 50 mcg of estrogen. If lower dosage preparations are used the LH and T.Te levels should be periodically checked to make sure that GN have really been reduced. The estrogenic profile of the "pill" can be obtained in different ways: by using only weakly androgenic progestins and by unbalancing the ratio and the doses of the steroid components. The use of associations with weakly androgenic progestins makes it possible to reduce the dose of estrogen without altering the estrogenic profile, thus inducing the SHBG increase and the consequent decrease of free blood androgens. The results we obtained (tab. 3) show that the treatment with this new monophasic combination (Diane-35®) can "normalize" the endocrine profile of PCOS and achieve a consequent improvement of clinical symptoms. The main and most important hormonal changes we observed during treatment were:

1. strong decrease of LH levels
2. drop of ovarian and adrenal androgens
3. strong increase of blood SHBG
4. decrease of F.Te blood values.

A significant LH drop can be seen already at the 6th treatment cycle follow-up examination and a further decrease in the absolute values can be seen at the 12th and 24th treatment cycle follow-up examinations. The decrease of LH and of the LH/FSH ratio at the 6th cycle must be considered effective because of the significant suppression of the ovarian hormones.

The following decrease of LH at the 12th cycle, together with the significant decrease of A and E_2 is also of great clinical importance because it proves the need to use this drug for more than 12 months in order to obtain the greatest therapeutic results. The significant decrease of DHEA-S shows the inhibition of the cortical adrenal activity induced by the association with CPA. The considerable decrease of SHBG confirms the effectivity of the EE dosage used in this new combination and partly explains the decrease of F.Te. PCOS is no doubt the most frequent cause of hirsutism in women. The main biological changes involved in determining the hyperandrogenism symptoms in PCOS are, on one hand, the increase in LH-induced androgen production, the decrease of SHBG and the binding capacity for blood T with increase of F.Te and consequent stimulation of the pilo-sebaceous unit. Even the DHEA-S that often increases in PCOS can contribute in the genesis of hyperandrogenism symptoms because at the peripheral level it can be converted to T and DHT. Therapy of hyperandrogenism must, therefore, reduce the ovarian-adrenal androgenic production, increase the SHBG synthesis, reduce the quota of blood F.Te and inhibit the conversion of A into compounds with a greater androgenic activity. In our study we showed how the new ethinyl estradiol/cyproterone acetate combination (Diane-35®) can achieve the aims required of an adequate therapy. In fact success percentages showed that the acne symptom disappeared in 100% of cases, seborrhea in 58%, and hirsutism in 66.7%.

The comparison between endocrine and clinical findings underlines the importance of the long term use (more than 1 year) of this new drug which has made PCOS therapy with low estrogen dosage and low incidence of side effects possible.

References

[1] Goldzieher, J. W., K. Elkind-Hirsch: Polycystic ovarian disease. New Trends Gyn. Obst. **1** (1985) 7.
[2] Givens, J. R., R. N. Andersen, W. L. Wiser et al.: Dynamics of suppression and recovery of plasma FSH LH Androstendione and Testosterone in Polycystic Ovarian Disease using an oral contraceptive. J. Clin. Endocrinol. Metab. **38** (1974) 727.
[3] Falsetti, L., D. Dordoni, C. Gastaldi et al.: A new association of ethinylestradiol (0.035 mg) cyproterone acetate (2 mg) in the therapy of polycystic ovary syndrome. Acta Europea Fertilitatis **17** (1986) 19.
[4] Wild, R. A., E. S. Umstot, R. N. Andersen et al.: Adrenal function in hirsutism. II Effect of an oral contraceptive, J. Clin. Endocrinol. Metab. **54** (1982) 676.
[5] Carr, B. R., C. R. Parker, J. D. Madden et al.: Plasma levels of adrenocorticotropin and cortisol in women receiving oral contraceptive steroid treatment. J. Clin. Endocrinol. Metab. **49** (1979) 346.
[6] Chang, R. J., F. P. Mandel, A. R. Wolfsen et al.: Circulating levels of plasma ACTH in Polycystic Ovarian Disease. J. Clin. Endocrinol. Metab. **54** (1982) 1256.
[7] Inaudi, P., G. D'Ambrogio, C. Massafra et al.: Impaired pregnenolone secretion after combined cyproterone acetate and ethynyl estradiol therapy in hirsute patients. Gynecol. Obstet. Invest. **14** (1982) 106—120.
[8] Lobo, R. A., O. A. Kletzky, G. S. Di Zerega: Elevated serum bioactive LH concentration in women with Polycystic Ovary Syndrom. Fertil. Steril. **37** (1982) 301.
[9] Raj, S. G., H. C. M. Raj, L. M. Talbert et al.: Normalization of plasma testosterone levels by low estrogen oral contraceptive in Polycystic Ovary Disease. Endocrine Society 63rd Annual Meeting, Cincinnati, Ohio, Program and Abstract, n. 452, 1981.
[10] Hammerstein, J., J. Meckies, I. Leo-Rossberg et al.: Use of cyproterone acetate (CPA) in the treatment of acne, hirsutism and virilism. J. Steroid. Biochem. **6** (1975) 827.
[11] Breckwoldt, M., R. Trolp, W. Braendle et al.: Antiandrogen oral contraceptives. In: International Symposium on Hormonal Contraception., Proc. Symp. Utrecht, 1977, 81. Excerpta Medica, Intern. Congress. Series 441, Amsterdam—Oxford 1978.
[12] Chapman, M. G., S. L. Jeffcoate, C. J. Dewhurst: Effect of Cyproterone acetate-etinylestradiol treatment on adrenal function in hirsute women. Clin. Endocrinol. **17** (1982) 577.

Discussion

Schindler: I want to open the discussion referring to the marvellous study of Prof. Falsetti and to his most interesting result, that there is a significant suppression of DHEAS, —a result, which Prof. Haspels mentioned already—; and I would like to ask Prof. Neumann, since he briefly pointed out the glucocorticoid effect of the antiandrogen cyproterone acetate, if he could delineate for us the effect of suppressing the ACTH levels according to the dose of cyproterone acetate.

Neumann: As I mentioned during my lecture there is no question, that in the usual labaratory animals like rats, guinea-pigs, hamster, cyproterone acetate and similar compounds like chlormadinone acetate or medroxyprogesterone acetate are able to suppress the pituitary-adrenal axis by inhibiting ACTH secretion and secondary inhibiting cortisol and corticosterone production. However, these animals never show any sign of secondary adrenal insufficiency. This is a very important point. Coming to the human situation we know from children treated for precosious puberty with dosis higher than 100—150 mg/qm that means a daily dose of 300—400 mg cyproterone acetate per child that only when given in such high dosis there is some suppression on the pituitary-adrenal-axis and the response of the adrenal during the ACTH test is reduced. But even though, these children never showed any signs of secondary adrenal insuffiency. Coming back to adult men and women, inspite of a great number of studies had been done, only a very few cases showed a reduced adrenal response during the treatment, which never was a clinical problem and a reason for stopping the treatment. But secondary adrenal insufficiency was also never observed even in high-dose treatment (300 mg/day) for instance used in patients treated for prostatic cancer or hypersexuality, some of them have been treated for more than 15 years contineously.

Schindler: Thank you very much for your clear comment. But I want to stress that I did not mean using cyproterone acetate would endanger the function of the hypothalamic-pituitary-adrenal-axis. I want to state this very clearly and I think this was your point you wanted to make. My point was another one. Based upon the results of the presentations of this morning sessions, —that you get a dramatic decrease of the circulating DHEAS, —I want to work out the following question.—Why do we get this dramatic decrease of DHEAS? Is that decrease a matter of suppression of the adrenal function, or also of ovarian function, or is this decrease an influence of this combination-preparation of an antiandrogen-estrogen directly or indirectly on the ovary in the first place and on the adrenal in the second place?

Neumann: There are two possibilities: First at least part of this DHEAS may be derived from the ovary—the hypothesis I want to prefer. The second possibility would be that adrenal androgen production is not so much under ACTH control as the synthesis of adrenal glucocorticoids.

Schindler: So you would say, that this is indeed an effect on the hypothalamic-pituitary-ovarian axis and at least not on the basis of ACTH suppression of the adrenal.

Spona: There is good agreement with that since also testosterone is reduced. There is no direct evidence, but it is certainly not the main point of action on the adrenal axis. I want to switch the subject to another point. There are some data in the literature showing that cyproterone acetate may have some intrinsic androgenic activity. We have shown in a lower dose range a weak androgenic action and in a higher dose range the antiandrogenic action. This biphasic action is similar to antiestrogens. Do you have similar data?

Falsetti: No. I have not.

Neumann: I want first to give the answer and then the explanation. The answer is clearly no. In all animal experiments we did, cyproterone acetate has no androgenic activity at any given dose. The most sensitive model for androgenicity is the female fetus. The femals fetus reacts very sensitive with virilization if the mother is treated during pregnancy, even if the compound has only a very little androgenicity. We have no evidence that this would be the case in animals and there is no evidence in human beings even at doses of up to 300 mg/daily.

Schindler: Thank you very much for your clear statement. So in conclusion I may repeat: Antiandrogens such as cyproterone acetate do not have any intrinsic androgenic action.

Now we still have open the first point of our discussion regarding the significant reduction of DHEAS under Diane-35® which has been shown clearly.

Gaspard (Belgium): I would like to bring a comparison with medroxyprogesterone acetate which by the way is closely related to cyproterone acetate. In that case there are some data indicating that medroxyprogesterone acetate has some intrinsic glucocorticoid action and it also reduces to some amount the level of circulating DHEAS.

Neumann: In which dose and for what indication did you use MPA?

Gaspard: 150 mg every 3 to 4 weeks for contraception intramuscularely.

Ermini (Rome): I want to note that the suppression of DHEAS is not only an effect on the ovary but also in the doses used a direct glucocorticoid effect of cyproterone acetate on the adrenal system. The zona reticularis is dependent on the LH stimulation. Diane-35® decreases LH which leads to a suppression of DHEAS not only of the ovary but also of the adrenal gland.

Schindler: Now we are at the point that we can unify the whole complex so far discussed: One can deduct from what has been said here—first of all the use of Diane-35® will cause a suppression of DHEAS from the ovary—however, from the doses used in this combination of an antiandrogen and an estrogen there is no direct glucocorticoid effect on the adrenal axis. Therefore taking in account the studies in pregnancy and you mentioned this that HCG, that is LH, is a stimulus for the zona reticularis, —that is the area of the adrenal which produces DHEAS—, we must consider that in all previous studies and in the study of Prof. Falsetti the high LH levels are decreased by Diane-35®. This is then resulting in a reduction of ovarian as well as adrenal production of DHEAS secretion via taking away the stimulus of LH.

Nürnberger: Was there any additional local theray for the acne or only the therapy with Diane-35®? I ask because of the very excellent results of Prof. Falsetti.

Falsetti: No, there was no additional treatment as far as I know.

Mrs. Aydinlik: Prof. Falsetti, do you have any experience whether after the cessation of therapy and the normalization of the hormonal parameters was there also an improvement in fertility?. Did your patients get pregnant?.

Falsetti: No, I would not be so hopeful, I think an additional treatment with clomiphene citrate is necessary.

Schindler: This is another important point which Mrs. Aydinlik just mentioned. There is another indication for using antiandrogenic therapy with cyproterone acetate/ethinyl estradiol combination which should however be considered with caution. In 1978 I published already a study with 100 mg cyproterone acetate and 40 µg EE in a reverse sequential manner, demonstrating that 33% improvement of cycle function after an average nine months treatment. Only 3% of the patients had worsening of menstrual cycle function after the treatment.

I think this leads us to a very important point in the discussion about the importance of Diane-35® in young women with signs of androgenization. Besides the clinical improvement of the signs of androgenization Diane-35® might have a prophylactic effect on future menstrual cycle function by changing the circulating androgen levels and their inhibiting effects on the female reproductive endocrine system. This is preventive gynecology in the best sense.

Neumann: I want to make a short comment. We are always looking at the androgen levels as a parameter of androgen deprivation. This is only one side of the coin and not the most important one. There is a dual mechanism of action, —one is the inhibition of gonadotropin secretion and inhibition of testosterone and androgen production, where ever this may be. But the second and most important one is the inhibition of androgens in the target organ. Of course, there is no possibility to measure the competition on the target organ but it is much more important than the inhibition or reduction of testosterone secretion.

Schindler: I thank you very much for your pointing out the cellular level. But as a clinician the clinical result is the most important matter: you get at least a side effect to be usefull later, namely the longterm improvement of the patients reproductive system using contraception on the one hand, using cycle regulation on the other hand and having an excellent systemic effect in regard of signs of androgenization.

Cohen: Would you suggest to use Diane-35® as a pretreatment in women with sterility problems comparable to the pretreatment of sterility patients with endometriosis?

Schindler: No, there is no indication for this type of patients for a pretreatment with Diane-35®. I was thinking about the young patients below 20 with signs of androgenization and giving Diane-35® with an outlook of simultanous improvement of signs of androgization and improving future menstrual cycle regulation.

Haspels: As clinicians we were all unhappy that chlormadinone acetate was taken out of the circulation due to the unsound FDA regulations. Don't you think, that chlormadinone acetate and cyproterone acetate—both are hydroxyprogesterone derivates—should be the first choice in general and preferable to 19-nortesterone derivates?

Schindler: When we talk about antiandrogenes today, and we compare cyproterone acetate with chlormadinone acetate from the clinical point of view, there is no question that cyproterone acetate is the first choice. This is because of the higher antiandrogenic effect per molecule of cyproterone acetate compared with chlormadinone acetate.

Neumann: Qualitatively the pattern of activity is almost identical comparing chlormadinone acetate and cyproterone acetate. But quantitatively cyproterone acetate is about 3 times more potent as an antiandrogen than chlormadinone acetate. There is also clinical evidence that cyproterone acetate containing preparations are superior to chlormadinone acetate preparations.

Schindler: From a clinical point of view I would fully agree with what Prof. Neumann said.

Haspels: Then you still could reduce the dose and use it in menopausal women in a lower dose. Therefore my question: Could it be preferable to nortestosterone preparations?

Schindler: You are raising now another important matter. If we talk about postmenopausal treatment and we consider gestagens and the comparison of 19-nortestosterone derivates and 17-alpha-hydroxyprogesterone derivates there is no question in my mind that we should prefer the progesterone derivatives. If there are signs of androgenization then we should also use a progesterone derivate with a stronger antiandrogenic effect. 19-nortestosterone preparation should not be used in postmenopausal treatment anymore.

Falsetti: Prof. Fedele, looking at your results of the effect of Diane-35® on the endometrium would you recommend this preparation also for premenopausal cyclic regulation?

Fedele: I think, the morphological changes with Diane-35® are very good. You see a reduction of hyperplastic lesions and especially no change in the small venules which leads to a very low rate of intermenstrual bleedings.

Schindler: Concerning postmenopausal substitution we talk of estradiol and cyproterone acetate. What are the morphological changes on that?

Fedele: We saw a reduction of the mucosa. We now have started a study of comparison of Diane-35®, Danazol and Gestrinon, but the data are not available.

Schindler: We want to get forward in our discussion and may I ask Prof. Haspels whether he could tell us his experiences how long the effect of antiandrogenic therapy will remain after treatment.

Haspels: This is very individual. About half of them will still remain improved for the next year and other will come back in three months and ask for the preparation because acne reappeared again.

Schindler: What is the experience in France with the combination of cyproterone acetate and the estrogel? Is there a longterm effect when taking the medication away?

Cohen: The experience with this combination was made by the group of Prof. Mauvais-Jarvis, especially by Mrs. Kutteen. Myself, I have no personel experience, but as far as I know from their results, they are very content with this combination.

Audebert: The only draw back of the combination of estrogel/cyproterone acetate is the individual variability of the absorption of the estrogel via the skin.

May I take the chance to ask Prof. Neumann regarding the antiestrogenic properties of cyproterone acetate which can be of advantage of the application in other indications?

Neumann: Of course the antiestrogenic potency of cyproterone acetate is some what less pronounced than with levonorgestrel, but it is present. Of course cyproterone acetate as a progestogene is also an antiestrogen. But your question was whether cyproterone acetate can be used for other indications, i.e. endometriosis and breast cancer. Principally yes, but only a very small clinical trial has been done in patients with prostatic carcinoma, but there do not exist any trial in endometriosis.

Lachnit: There ist very limited experience with cyproterone acetate for the treatment of endometriosis. A very preliminary trial was done in Munich with a daily dose of 10 mg cyproterone acetate and they have some favourable impression, but this was no control study.

Schindler: I just want to make a comment. A daily dose of 10 mg cyproterone acetate is an insufficient therapy the same as with the same dose of lynestrenol.

Haspels: You need at least 50 mg cyproterone acetate/day, because you have to get them amenorrhoic.

Schindler: Thank you very much. I absolutely agree with you on this point.

We still have one point open, which I do not want to miss, since we have two speakers who presented their data on ovulation inhibition effect. Prof. Spona and Prof. Hutchinson would you like to comment on that.

I think the presentation of Dr. Hutchinson has clearly shown that when you change from one preparation to the other there is no danger that there might be unvoluntary ovulation.

Hutchinson: Yes, in all patients there was no ovulation.

Schindler: Prof. Spona pointed out that there is no ovulation on the basis of progesterone measurements, however there is the possibility of follicular development. I would like to ask him to make a comment on this.

Spona: One has to stress that follicular maturation can be seen in all low dose preparations, also observed by ultrasonic investigations. In our data LH and FSH levels measured at day 5 of the cycle were very high indicating that follicular maturation has occured during the intervall between stopping the pill and starting the medication again. It is of interest that this phenomen takes place after the first two treatment cycles and could not be visualized during the first two treatment cycles. But no ovulation occured, so that it is a safe oral contraceptive preparation.

Gaspard: I like to fully support the answer of Prof. Spona. In our extensive ultrasonic studies on low dose pill takers we saw in a subset of patients of about 15 to 20% during the first days of the new cycle the development of follicles, which can develop up to 10 to 12 mm for a short period of time about 5 to 6 days. In the control ultrasonic scan on day 11 or 12 of the cycle the follicular structure has completely disappeared in all patients.

Schindler: Ladies and Gentlemen. To summarize I want to make a final comment. First I want to console Prof. Spona because of his one patient where he found a discrepancy of the E2 levels and the LH and FSH. I think there is no discrepancy what so ever. He obtains the suppression of LH and FSH because E2 rises. Second I would like to thank all the speakers and all the discussants in particular because I think we had a lively and successful discussion.

III Effects on the haemostatic system

Longitudinal study on the effects of a cyproterone acetate and ethinyl estradiol combination on haemostasis

V. Bruni, S. Bucciantini, D. Rosati, A. Verni, R. Abbate, S. Pinto

Introduction

The use of cyproterone acetate (CPA) in the treatment of acne vulgaris is now an effective therapy. Even though acne vulgaris cannot be considered an endocrine disease, it has been demostrated definitively that androgens are an essential factor in the development of acne. In fact, the pilosebaceous unit is an androgen end organ, and sebum secretion is principally induced by androgens.

Increased androgenic activity can be induced in two ways [3]:

1. By an enhanced amount of circulating androgens due to increased ovarian or adrenal production
2. By a stronger reaction of end-organ to normal androgen levels. An altered cutaneous androgen metabolism with formation of more potent metabolites can take place: patients with acne show an increased conversion of testosterone to DHT by 5 α-reductase in the skin [8].

The cyproterone acetate, because of its active mechanism (competition with the 5 α-DHT citoplasmic and nuclear receptors), can be considered particularly effective in dealing with both of these occurences. The combination with ethinyl estradiol, besides augmenting the binding capacity of testosterone to its protein carrier, diminishes the level of free testosterone and arrests the secretion of ovarian androgens.

As do all other estrogen-progestin combinations, ethinyl estradiol/cyproterone acetate causes some side-effects. Of notable interest are the possible repercussions on the haemostatic system particularly evident with combinations of high estrogen-progestin content.

Materials and methods

We have investigated the effects of a treatment with a new low-dose antiandrogenic combination of 35 mcg ethinyl estradiol and 2 mg cyproterone acetate on the haemostatic system. The study was performed longitudinally in 20 healthy subjects aged 18—35 years (average 23,4). Platelet functions (platelet aggregate ratio, beta-thromboglobulin, and megathrombocyte count), blood coagulation (fibrinopeptide A and antithrombin III) and fibrinolytic activity (resting and after stimulation) were investigated before and after 1, 3, 6, and 9 cycles of treatment.

Throughout the study no significant changes were observed in platelet functions. Platelet and megathrombocyte count showed no changes during the treatment. Circulating platelet aggregate amount (fig. 1) and beta-thromboglobulin production (fig. 1) did not change significantly.

FPA concentration (fig. 2) remained unchanged after 1 cycle, but increased by at least 1 ng/ml in 13 out of the 20 subjects after 3 cycles. The mean values increased from 1.3 ± 0.42 ng/ml to 2.8 ± 1.72 ng/ml ($p < 0.001$), 6% of values recorded at this time were out of the normal range of baseline values (mean + 2

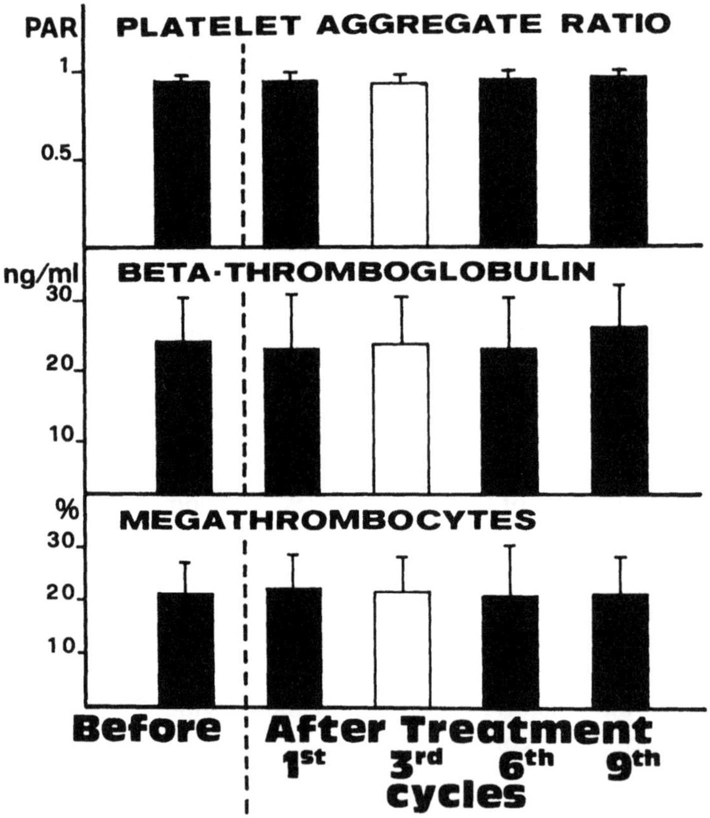

Fig. 1 Platelet aggregate ratio, beta-thromboglobulin and megathrombocytes before and after treatment. Platelet and megathrombocyte count was performed in whole blood by Platelet Analyzer 810 (Baker Instruments, Allentown PA, USA). Platelet aggregate ratio was investigated according to Wu and Hoak [12]. Beta-thromboglobulin was assayed by R.I.A., according to Ludlam [11].

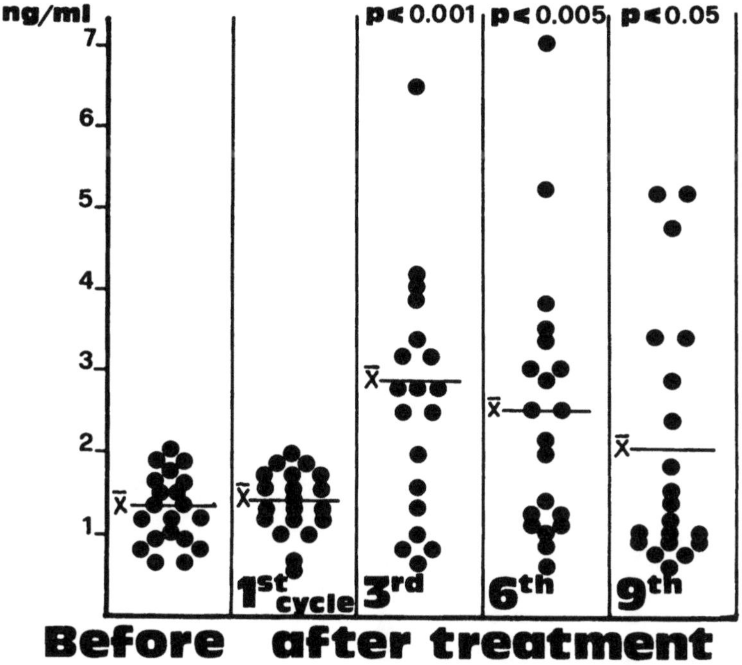

Fig. 2 Fibrinopeptide A concentration before and after treatment. FPA was measured in platelet poor plasma by R.I.A. according to Hofmann and Straub [9].

standard deviations). After 6 cycles mean FPA concentration was significantly higher (2.48 ± 1.6 ng/ml) than that before the beginning of the treatment, but lower than after 3 cycles. 50% of the values were out of the normal range of baseline values. After 9 cycles of treatment, FPA concentration (2.0 ± 1.56 ng/ml) was still higher than before treatment, but a further decrease occurred in 80% of subjects and only 7 out of the 20 subjects (35%) were out of the normal range.

AT III activity (fig. 3) showed slight, but statistically significant, changes during treatment. After the first cycle, a tendency toward a slight, but not significant, decrease was observed. However, after the third cycle the values of AT III activity were not different from basal values. After subsequent cycles, a steady, statistically significant increase was observed. In fact, after the first 6 cycles mean values increased from 100.5 ± 9.21% to 124.4 ± 15.36%. The increase was observed in 13 of 20 subjects (65%). After 9 cycles the increase was found in 16 of 20 subjects (80%).

All subjects but one (fig. 4) were called "good responders" as they showed a doubling of fibrinolytic activity after stimulation. As far as the effects of treatment are concerned, no alterations of resting fibrinolytic activity were found throughout the study. Fibrinolytic response was found significantly increased after 6 cycles 17.7 ± 6.36 F.U. ($p < 0.025$) and after 9 cycles 17.3 ± 4.5 F.U.

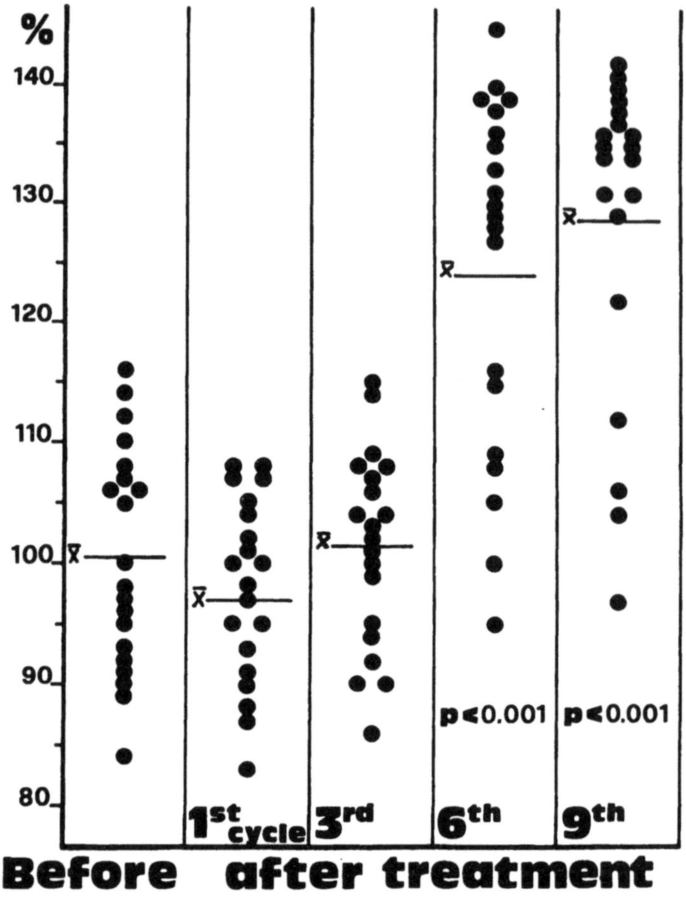

Fig. 3 Antithrombin III activity before and after treatment. AT III activity was measured according to Abildgaard et al. [1].

($p < 0.01$) in comparison to pre-treatment values (13.2 ± 6.3 F.U.). Routine blood clotting tests showed significant changes throughout the study.

Conclusions

The observed estro-progestin combination demonstrated absence of platelet activation "in vivo" during the course of 9 cycles of treatment. Coagulation activation, documented by the increase of FPA, is present after the 3rd cycle, but tends to diminish progressively after the 6th and 9th cycles of treatment.

The above-mentioned activation is also accompanied by an activation of coagulation inhibitors as determined through the study of AT III, which is one of the principal inhibitors of the coagulation process.

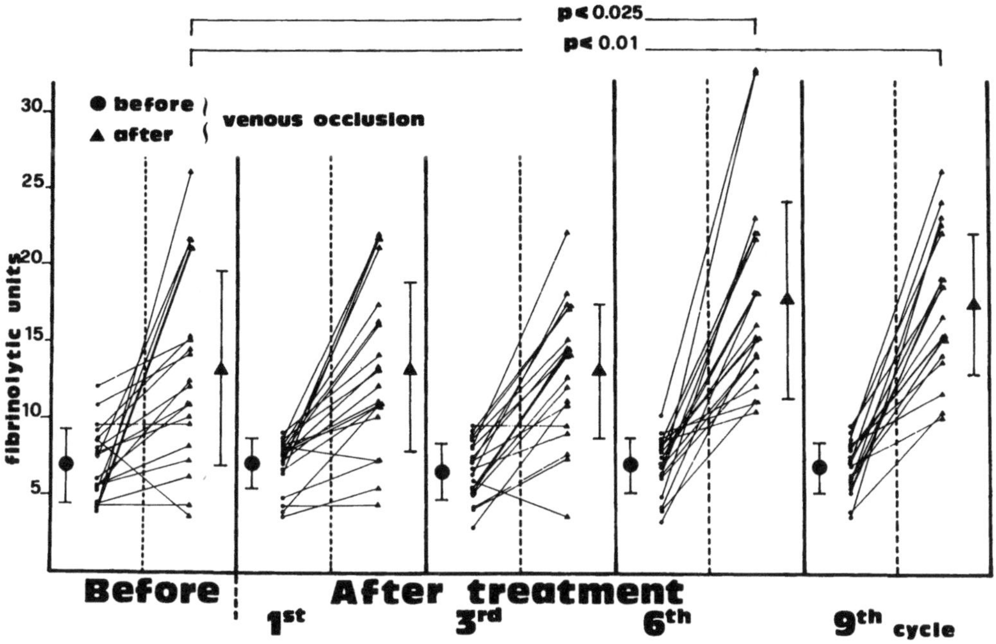

Fig. 4 Fibrinolytic activity (• before and ▲ after venous occlusion). Spontaneous plasma fibrinolytic activity was assayed by Euglobulin Clot Lysis Time, according to Januszko and Dubinska [10]. Fibrinolytic potential was determined by forearm venous occlusion, (15 min. occlusion, cuff pressure 10 mmHg below DBP) for the assessment of the release of plasminogen activator from vessel wall.

Slight but significant increase of fibrinolysis was observed after the 6th and 9th cycle of treatment. This combination, which is particularly indicated in cases of slight hyperandrogenism, causes some effects on the haemostatic system; these effects are, however, clearly less significant than those of formulations with higher doses of either ethinyl estradiol or cyproterone acetate.

Hammerstein [6] reported a 1% incidence of thrombophlebitis after the administration of 50 mcg ethinyl estradiol in combination with 100 mg of cyproterone acetate a day for at least 3 cycles as part of a wide-range study of 602 patients. This percentage goes down to 0.53% in a case-study of 188 women treated with the combined therapy using the same dose of ethinyl estradiol but a lower dose (2 mg) of cyproterone acetate.

In a former study [4] on the effects of the reverse sequential therapy with cyproterone acetate and ethinyl estradiol on 12 subjects from the ages of 17 through 34, we of the Department of Obstretrics and Gynecology of the University of Florence have proven a significant activation of the haemostatic system as shown by the increase of circulating platelet aggregates (fig. 5) and by the increase of soluble fibrinic complexes already present after the 1st month

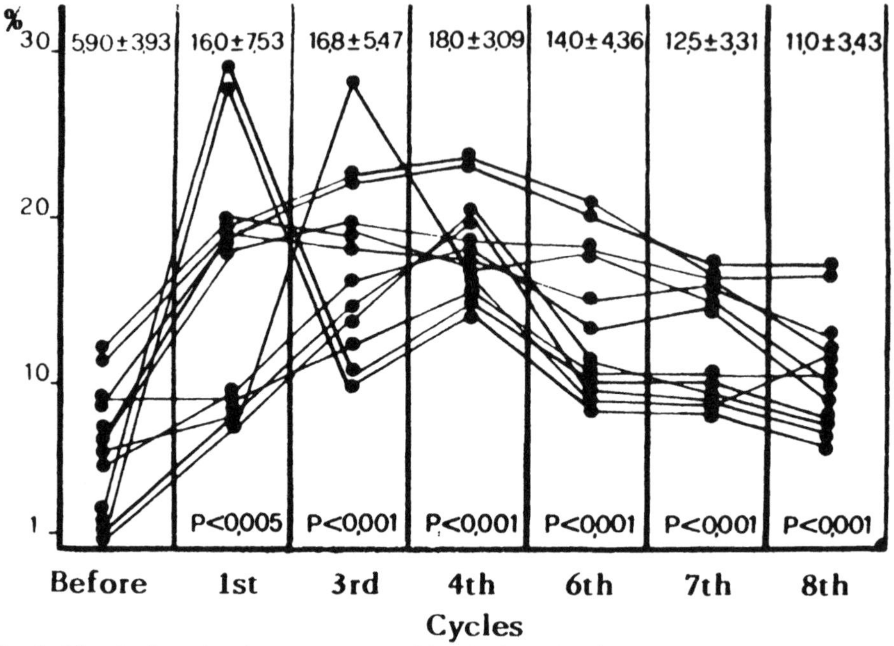

Fig. 5 Circulating platelet aggregates. Circulating platelet aggregates were analysed according to Wu and Hoak [12].

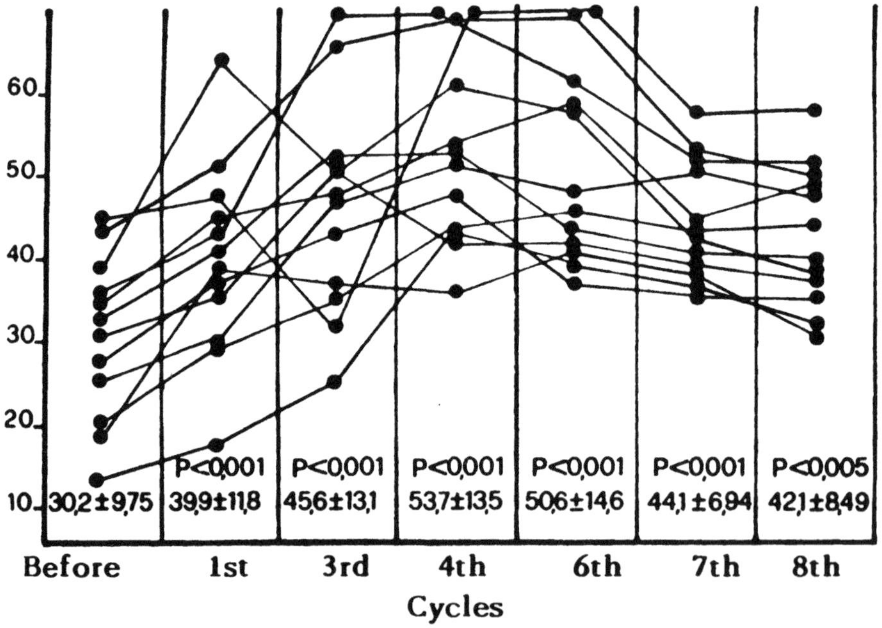

Fig. 6 Soluble fibrin complex. Soluble fibrin complex was analysed by fibrinogen gel chromatography, according to Hafter and Greed [7].

(fig. 6). Moreover, a reduction of fibrinolytic potential after venous occlusion was present in all the observed cycles (fig. 7).

Many reseachers have demonstrated modifications favorable to coagulation during the treatment with the combination of ethinyl estradiol 50 mcg and cyproterone acetate 2 mg. These were accompanied by a slight increase of the fibrinolytic activity. Moreover, the parallel activation of the antithrombotic mechanisms (AT III and the fibrinolysis) in absence of platelet activation contributes to the re-establishment of the haemostatic balance.

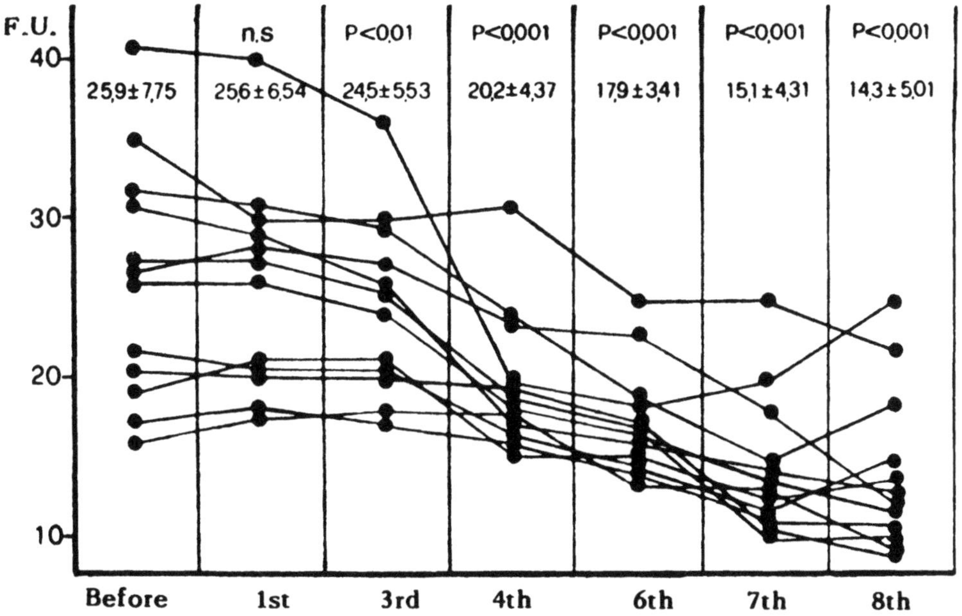

Fig. 7 Fibrinolytic potential after venous occlusion (15 min. occlusion, Cuff pressure 10 mmHg below DPB) was measured by Euglobulin Clot Lysis time [10].

References

[1] Abilgaard, U., K. Gravem, H. C. Godal: Assay of progressive antithrombin in plasma. Thromb. Dath. Haemorrh. **24** (1970) 224.

[2] Aydinlik, S., U. Lachnit-Fixson: Diane – eine Gestagen-Oestrogen Kombination mit Antiandrogenwirkung. Med. Monatsschr. **31** (1979) 425.

[3] Darley, C. R., J. D. Kirby, G. M. Besser et al.: Circulating testosterone, sex hormone binding globulin and prolactin in women with late onset or persistent acne vulgaris. Brit. J. of Dermatology **106** (1982) 517.

[4] Gasparri, F., V. Bruni, M. Dei et al.: Impiego clinico del ciproterone acetato. In: Bompiani, A., N. Garcea (eds.): Argomenti di sterilità. Atti del X Congr. Soc. It. Fertil. Steril. p. 105, 1980.

[5] Gezzo, F., C. Manieri, R. Rodi et al.: Effects of the cyproterone acetate + Ethynil-Oestradiol antiandrogen association on blood coagulation and fibrinolysis in hirsute women. Panminerva medica **23**, 4 (1981) 223.
[6] Hammerstein, J.: Antiandrogene. Arch. Gynäkol. **214** (1973) 243.
[7] Hafter, R., H. Greed: Molecular aspect of defibrination in a reptilase-treated case of dead fetus syndrome. Thromb. Res. **7** (1975) 391.
[8] Hay, J. B., M. B. Hodgins: Metabolism of androgens by human skin in acne. Brit. J. of Dermatology **91** (1974) 123.
[9] Hofmann, V., P. W. Straub: A radioimmunoassay technique for the rapid measurement of human fibrinopeptide A. Throm. Res. **11** (1977) 171.
[10] Januszko, I., L. Dubinska: Estimation of the activator of the fibrinolysis by means of the euglobulin test. Acta Med. Polona **6** (1965) 269.
[11] Ludlam, C. A.: Evidence for the platelet specificity of beta-thromboglobulin and studies of its plasma concentrations in healthly individuals. Brit. J. Haemat. **41** (1979) 271.
[12] Wu, K. K., J. C. Hoak: A new method for the quantitative detection of platelet aggregates in patients with arterial insufficiency. Lancet **II** (1974) 923.

Haemorheological effects of Diane-35® and Microgynon® — Preliminary results of a double blind study

E. Ernst, Ch. Schmölzl, A. Matrai, W. Schramm

Introduction

There have repeatedly been epidemiological reports suggesting that oral contraceptives increase the risk of cardiovascular diseases [27, 28, 29, 34]. In particular, brain and heart infarction and venous thromboembolism seem to be more frequent in women taking the pill [21, 32, 33]. The underlying biological mechanisms hypothesised to explain this vary from alterations in lipid and carbohydrate metabolism [25, 30], increase in blood pressure, to changes in the coagulation system [20]. Yet another possible factor might be the rheology of blood [12]. It has been shown that the flow properties of blood (quantifiable ex vivo by measuring haematocrit, blood and plasma viscosity as well as blood cell filterability) are intimately related to cardiovascular risk factors and diseases [8, 13]. Moreover, several investigators (tab. 1) have demonstrated that the

Table 1 Overview of studies on oral contraception and blood rheology

first author type of study	n	type	medication estrogen	gestagen	results
Aronson/L	25/22	S/O	E	M/NA	(Hk ↑), (BV ↑)
Oski/CS	34	O	?	?	RCD ↓
Durocher/CS	20	?	?	?	no change
Leonhardt/CS	15	?	?	?	(BV ↑), PV ↑
Leonhardt/CS	33	?	?	?	(BV ↑)
Lowe/CS	25	?	?	?	Hk ↑, BV ↑, Fib ↑
Easthope/CS	11	?	?	?	no change
Brooks/L	?	?	?	?	Fib ↑
Buchan/CS	38	O	E	N	Hk ↑, (BV ↑), (PV ↑), (RDC ↓), (FIB ↑)
Heilman/CS	11/22	S/O	E	N	(Hk ↓), BV ↑, RCD ↓

CS = cross-sectional, L = longitudinal, S = sequential, O = one phase, E = ethinyl estradiol, M = medroxyprogesterone, NA = norethisteronacetat, N = norgestrel, Hk = haematocrit, BV = blood viscosity, RDC = red cell deformability, PV = plasma viscosity, Fib = fibrinogen
( ) unter certain conditions only

rheology of blood is adversely affected by oral contraception [1, 2, 4, 6, 7, 15, 17, 18, 19, 26]. The aim of the present study was, therefore, to test in a controlled double-blind trial, whether the medication of relatively low-dose hormonal contraceptives influence haemorheological variables.

Materials and methods

Subjects

50 female volunteers aged 20—30 years were admitted into the trial. Exclusion criteria were body weight more than 10% in excess of normal, abnormal gynaecological findings (including cytology and palpation of mammae), contraindications for oral contraception, pregnancy, any long term medication, short term medication using drugs interacting with oral contraceptives, hypertension, diabetes, consumption of more than 10 cigarettes or 40 ml alcohol per day.

Study design

The trial started with a phase of no hormones lasting for 3 cycles. In the third cycle blood was taken three times (between days 1—8, 13—15, and 24—28). Subsequently the volunteers were randomized into group A or B. Group A took Diane-35® (0.035 mg ethinyl estradiol and 2.0 mg cyproterone acetate), group B Microgynon® (0.03 mg ethinyl estradiol and 0.15 mg levonorgestrel) for 6 cycles. 2 weeks after starting the medication a pregnancy was excluded by immunological testing (Pregslide®). During the medication phase blood was taken at the end (between day 15—21) of the first, third, and sixth cycle. Finally

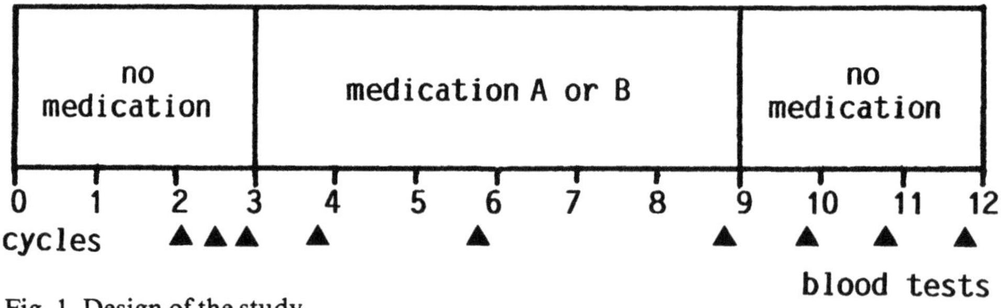

Fig. 1 Design of the study.
Legend:
The trial lasted for 12 cycles. After 3 cycles without medication, women were randomized into medication groups A or B. The following part of the study was double blind. The medication lasted for 6 cycles. It was followed by 3 cycles without medication. Whenever tests were run, this is shown by ▲.

a phase of no medication followed. It lasted 3 cycles, and blood was taken at day 21— 24 of each of these cycles. The study design is illustrated in figure 1.

Experimental methods

Blood sampling was performed after the subject had sat quietly for 10 min. An antecubital vein was punctured with a 21G butterfly and blood was drawn with minimal suction and no venous occlusion, a technique which excludes sampling artifacts [10]. Within 2 hours of withdrawl the following tests were performed in duplicate or triplicate:

- native blood viscosity at 37°C and defined shear rates (LS 30 Contraves) [31]
- blood viscosity as above at haematocrit of 45% [22]
- haematrocrit (microhaematrocrit centrifuge)
- plasma viscosity at 37°C (Coulter Harkness) [14]
- colloid oncotic pressure of plasma (Osmomat, Gonotec) [9]
- blood cell filterability (5 μm Nuclepore) [5]

Statistics

An analysis of co-variance was performed to evaluate differences between groups A and B using the mean values of the third blood test as a co-variable. For the longitudinal comparisons the Wilcoxon test for paired data was applied. The null-hypothesis was rejected when p was less than 0.05.

Results

Cross-sectional comparison

After three cycles of medication the native blood viscosity at low and middle shear rate as well as the plasma viscosity are higher in group B than in group A (tab. 2). In addition, all other haemorheological variables show that blood fluidity is slightly but not significantly decreased in group B at this point. At the last cycle of medication the plasma viscosity is still higher in group B. However, at the same time, the high shear blood viscosity at 45% haematocrit is significantly lower in this group. Here again, the native blood viscosity reveals a non-significant tendency to be higher in group B. At the end of the trial period there is a significant difference in the low shear native blood viscosity between groups A and B.

Table 2 Cross-sectional comparison: Haemorheological differences between group A and B (adjusted mean values)

parameter	dimension	last test in 3rd cycle	test in 6th cycle		test in 9th cycle		test in 12th cyle	
		group A and B	group A	group B	group A	group B	group A	group B
Haematocrit	%	39.9	38.7	39.7	39.0	40.7	40.5	40.9
Blood viscosity D = 0.7 s−1	mPa s	18.8	17.8	20.6*	19.9	20.7	18.7	20.9*
Blood viscosity D = 2.4 s−1	mPa s	10.9	10.5	11.6*	11.2	11.5	10.9	11.8
Blood viscosity D = 94.5 s−1	mPa s	4.1	4.1	4.2	4.1	4.1	4.1	4.2
Blood viscosity (45) D = 0.7 s−1	mPa s	27.0	27.7	30.3	33.5	27.5	25.7	27.7
Blood viscosity (45) D = 2.4 s−1	mPa s	14.6	15.1	15.6	17.1	14.4	14.2	14.7
Blood viscosity (45) D = 94.5 s−1	mPa s	4.9	5.0	5.0	5.1	4.7*	4.7	4.8
Plasma viscosity	mPa s	1.17	1.17	1.19*	1.17	1.20*	1.17	1.18
blood cell filterability	units	0.76	0.78	0.76	0.80	0.78	0.76	0.76

D = shear rate (45) = at haematocrit of 45% * = significant difference between A and B

Longitudinal comparisons

Table 3 shows longitudinal comparisons in which the values of each group are compared to its last baseline values (blood test No. 3). In the group treated with Diane-35® there is no significant deterioration of blood fluidity. On the contrary, the changes of native blood viscosity at high shear rate and blood cell filterability suggest an increase in fluidity. In the Microgynon®-treated group a significant increase in low and middle shear blood viscosity during medication can be seen. Plasma viscosity is elevated throughout the medication period, and there is a transient rise in low and middle shear blood viscosity at 45% haematocrit, which occurred after 3 months of medication. Figure 2 illustrates the box plots for plasma viscosity which are representative for most of the other results.

Table 3 Longitudinal comparisons: Haemorheological changes during medication A and B

parameter	dimension	medication A			medication B		
		test in 4th cycle	test in 6th cycle	test in 9th cycle	test in 4th cycle	test in 6th cycle	test in 9th cycle
Haematocrit	%	1.0	1.0	1.0	0.0	−1.0	0.0
Blood viscosity D = 0.7 s−1	mPa s	−0.6	1.4	−0.8	−2.8*	−1.9*	−2.3*
Blood viscosity D = 2.4 s−1	mPa s	−0.4	0.7	−0.3	−1.0*	−0.9	−0.7*
Blood viscosity D = 94.5 s−1	mPa s	−0.04	0.1*	0.06	−0.1	−0.1	−0.03
Blood viscosity (45) D = 0.7 s−1	mPa s	−0.8	−2.8	−3.0	−2.1	−2.8*	−1.6
Blood viscosity (45) D = 2.4 s−1	mPa s	−0.4	−0.5	−1.0	−1.2	−0.8*	−0.3
Blood viscosity (45) D = 94.5 s−1	mPa s	−0.1	−0.1	0.1	−0.1	−0.1	0.1
Plasma viscosity	mPa s	−0.01	0.01	0.0	−0.03*	−0.03*	−0.03*
Blood cell filterability	units	0.0	−0.04	−0.06*	0.03	0.04	0.0

Abbreviations as in tab. 2.
The mean differences of baseline (test No. 3) and tests during medication are shown, hence negative values indicate an increase compared to baseline.

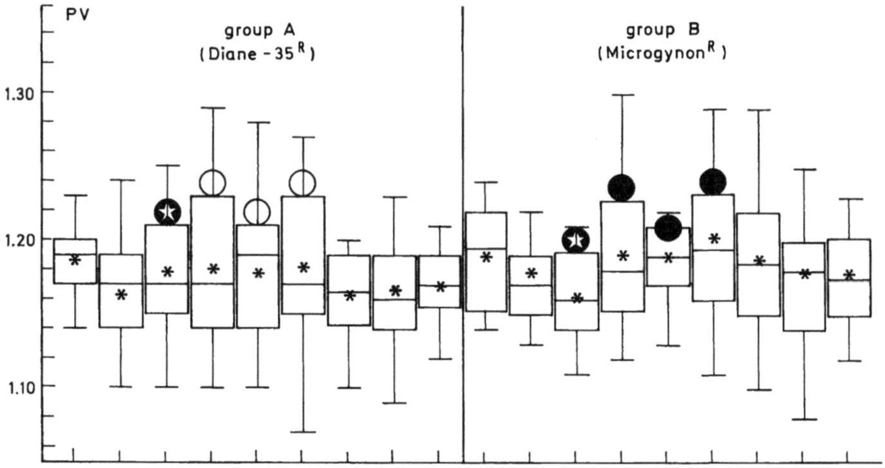

Fig. 2 Plasma viscosity in group A and B

Legend: Plasma viscosity in mPa s (vertical axis) illustrated by box plots as a function of time. Each box plot represents one measuring point as outlined in fig. 1. Significance was tested between the 3rd value of 3rd cycle ✪ and values during therapy.

● = significant change ○ = no significant change

Discussion

The present findings suggest that no changes of blood fluidity occur in women taking Diane-35® and some slight alterations take place in women taking Microgynon®. Theoretically it is possible that the time factor has introduced an artifact into the longitudinal study. There is no reason, however, why this should have happened selectively in group B, as both groups were studied parallelly. No significant deterioration of blood fluidity is seen in group A. Hence this possibility is an unlikely explanation for our findings.

In the cross-sectional comparison significant differences between the two medications were found. All except one (high shear blood viscosity at haematocrit 45% in the last cycle of medication) indicated that blood fluidity is lower in the Microgynon®-treated women. This is particularly true for plasma viscosity, which is the variable with the least methodological and biological variation [11]. In other words, both the longitudinal and the cross-sectional analysis suggest no changes due to Diane-35® and a slight, but significant decrease of blood fluidity due to Microgynon®. This suggests that the differences in the non-estrogen component of the two formulations influence the fluidity of blood. There is some epidemological evidence supporting the view that high progestagen activity may lead to higher incidences in arterial disease [16, 23, 24]. Most older studies on oral contraceptives and blood rheology show more pronounced haemorheological changes than the present one. However, in the majority of these trials the dosage and types of hormones were not defined. It is likely that the average hormone dose used then was higher than that in Diane-35® or Microgynon®. Possibly estrogen and progesterone activities exert differing effects on blood rheology. This view is supported by one study in which 1×0.05 mg/day ethinyl estradiol and 3×5 mg norethisteron were tested separately [3]. Both substances induced an increase in haematocrit and blood viscosity when taken for 3 months. The first, however, led to an increase, while the second induced a decrease in blood cell filterability. Diane-35® and Microgynon® have a similar estrogen component and progestagen activity, but Microgynon® has some androgenic potential while Diane-35® does not. One could therefore speculate that the haemorheological effects of Microgynon® might be caused by the androgenic activity of the drug. Clearly more work is needed to differentiate between various hormonal effects on blood rheology.

Finally, the duration of medication needs to be taken into consideration. In the reports in the literature mentioned above [1, 2, 4, 6, 7, 15, 17, 18, 19, 26] this factor is almost invariably undefined. In most trials it was 3 months or longer. Therefore, the literature suggests that oral contraceptives may lead to limitations in blood fluidity when administered at relatively high doses for prolonged periods of time. Our results imply that Dinae-35® taken for 6 months has no negative effects on blood rheology. Microgynon®, in contrast, induces some slight, but significant rheological changes. Whether these are involved in an increase of cardiovascular complications is debatable.

Summary

The hypothesis that oral contraceptives influence haemorheological variables is supported by a number of published studies. Since such effects might be relevant for cardiovascular complications associated with the pill, a controlled study was undertaken. 50 women were randomised into group A or B. Both groups were left without medication for 3 months. Subsequently they took either Diane-35® (A) or Microgynon® (B) for 6 months. This was followed by 3 months with no medication. Blood rheology was quantified 9 times by measuring blood and plasma viscosity, haematocrit, blood cell filterability, and plasma colloid oncotic pressure. The results show no significant changes in group A. In group B there was a significant rise in blood and plasma viscosities during medication. Cross-sectional comparisons between groups A and B reveal differences suggestive of decreased blood fluidity in group B. It is concluded that Diane-35®, taken for 6 months, does not induce relevant haemorheological alterations, while Microgynon® seems to lead to a slight but significant limitation of blood fluidity.

References

[1] Aronson, H. B., F. Magora, J. G. Schenker: Effect of oral contraceptives on blood viscosity. Amer. J. Obstet. Gynec. **110** (1971) 997—1001.

[2] Brooks, D. E.: Oral contraception: consequences for blood rheology and related parameters. Clin. Hemorheol. **1,** 3 (1981) 302—303.

[3] Buchan, P. C.: Haemorheological consequences of oestrogen and progestagen therapy. Int. J. Microcirc. Clin. Exp. **1** (1982) 262.

[4] Buchan, P. C., H. N. Mac Donald: Altered hemorheology in oral-contraceptive users. Br. Med. J. **I** (1980) 978—979.

[5] Dodds, A. J., P. Flute, J. Dormandy et al.: Haemorheological response to plasma exchange in Raynaud Syndrome. Brit. Med. J. **2** (1979) 1186.

[6] Durocher, J. R., M. S. Weir, E. G. Lundblad et al.: Effect of oral contraceptives and pregnancy on erythrocyte deformability and surface charge. Proceedings of the Society for Experimental Biology and Medicine **150** (1975) 368—370.

[7] Easthope, P. L., D. E. Brooks: A comparison of rheological constitutive functions for whole human blood. Biorheology **17** (1980) 235—247.

[8] Ernst, E.: Hämorheologie für den Praktiker, S. 42—45, 30—40. W. Zuckschwerdt Verlag München, Bern, Wien 1986.

[9] Ernst, E., A. Matrai: Messung des kolloidosmotischen Druckes. Labor Praxis **20** (1984) Nov.

[10] Ernst, E., A. Matrai: Pitfalls of blood sampling. Haematologica **71** (1986) 195—199.

[11] Ernst, E., A. Matrai, A. Scherer et al.: Methodological and intra-individual variations in some hemorheological tests. Clin. Hemorheol. **5** (1985) 511—514.

[12] Ernst, E., Ch. Schmölzl, A. Matrai: Koronarsklerose und Herzinfarkt bei jungen Frauen. Münch. Med. Wschr. **127** (1985) 13.

[13] Ernst, E., T. Weihmayr, M. Schmid et al.: Cardiovascular risk factos and hemorheology. Physical fitness, stress and obesity. Atherosclerosis **59** (1986) 263—269.

[14] Harkness, J.: A new method for the measurement of plasma viscosity. Lancet **2** (1963) 280.

[15] Heilmann, L., P. F. Tauber, U. Siekmann et al.: Die Fließfähigkeit des Blutes unter Einnahme von Ovulationshemmern. Zbl. Gynäkol. **103** (1981) 678—686.

[16] Kay, R.: Progesteron and arterial disease—Evidence from the Royal College of General Practitioneers' study. Am. J. Obstet. Gynecol. **142** (1982) 762—765.

[17] Leonhardt, H., H. G. Grigoleit, I. Reinhardt: Auswirkungen von Zigarettenrauch und oralen Kontrazeptiva auf die Plasma- und Vollblutviskosität. Med. Wel **29** (1978) 880—883.

[18] Leonhardt, H., A. Uthoff, I. Stelter: Veränderungen der Blut- und Plasmaviskosität bei Patienten mit Risikofaktoren. Med. Klin. **70** (1975) 1997—2000.

[19] Lowe, G. D. O., M. M. Drummond, C. D. Forbes et al.: Increased blood viscosity in young women using oral contraceptives. Am. J. Obstet. Gynecol. **137** (1980) 840—842.

[20] Mammen, E. F.: Oral contraceptives and blood coagulation: A critical review. Am. J. Obstet. Gynecol. **142** (1982) 781—790.

[21] Mann, J. I.: Progestogens in cardiovascular disease: An introduction to the epidemiologic data. Am. J. Obstet. Gynecol. **142** (1982) 752—757.

[22] Matrai, A., P. T. Flute, J. Dormandy: Improving accuracy of co-axial viscometry. Biorheology suppl. **1** (1984) 99.

[23] Meade, T. W.: Effects of progestrogens on the cardiovascular system. Am. J. Obstet. Gynecol. **142** (1982) 776—780.

[24] Meade, T. W., G. Greenberg, S. G. Thompson: Progestogens and cardiovascular reactions associated with oral contraceptives and a comparison of the safety of 50- and 30 μg oestrogen preparations. Brit. Med. J. **280** (1980) 1157—1161.

[25] Merians, D. R., W. L. Haskell, K. M. Vranizan et al.: Relationship of exercise, oral contraceptive use and body fat to concentrations of plasma lipids and lipoprotein cholesterol in young women. Am. J. Med. **78** (1985) 913—919.

[26] Oski, F. A., B. Lubin, E. Dober Buchert: Reduced red cell filterability with oral contraceptive agents. Annals of Internal Medicine **77** (1972) 417—419.

[27] Petitti, D. B., J. Wingerd, F. Pellegrin et al.: Risk of vascular disease in women: smoking, oral contraceptives, noncontraceptive estrogens and other factors. JAMA **242** (1979) 1150—1154.

[28] Royal College of General Practitioners: Mortality among oralcontraceptive users. Lancet **a/I** (1977) 727—731.

[29] Royal College of General Practitioners: Effect on hypertension and benign breast disease of progestagen component in combined oral contraceptives. Lancet **II** (1977) 624.

[30] Spellacy, W. N.: Carbohydrate metabolism during treatment with estrogen, progestogen and low-dose oral contraceptives. Am. J. Obstet. Gynecol. **142** (1982) 732—734.

[31] Spinelli, F. R., Ch. D. Meier: Measurement of blood viscosity. Biorheology **11** (1974) 301.

[32] Stadel, B. V.: Oral contraceptives and cardiovascular disease (second of two parts). N. Engl. J. Med. **305** (1981) 672—677.

[33] Stadel, B. V.: Oral contraceptives and cardiovascular disease (first of two parts). N. Engl. J. Med. **305** (1981) 612—618.

[34] Vessey, M. P., K. McPherson, B. Johnson: Mortality among women participating in the Oxford Family Planning Association contraceptive study. Lancet **I** (1977) 731—733.

Antiandrogen treatment in women with acne: a controlled trial

R. E. Ashton, J. A. Miller, F. T. Wojnarowska, P. M. Dowd, T. J. O'Brien, W. A. D. Griffiths, H. S. Jacobs

Introduction

Acne is known to be androgen dependent and in women responds to antiandrogen therapy. The etiology of acne is unknown but several factors play a part. Sebum excretion rate (SER) correlates well with the severity of the acne [5] and is androgen dependent [15]. Androgens also affect the disturbed keratinization of the follicle infundibulum [16].

Cyproterone acetate (CPA) is an antiandrogen which competes with dihydrotestosterone for the peripheral androgen receptor [14], and inhibits the translocation of the hormone receptor complex into the cell nucleus [3]. Both reduction in sebum excretion rate and clinical improvement of acne occur after treatment with large doses of estrogen [12]. Combined oral contraceptives (O/C) contain a maximum of 50 μg of estrogen, but even treatment with this dose results in a reduction of SER [13].

The most effective hormonal combination in the treatment of acne seems to be the combination of estrogen with the antiandrogen cyproterone acetate which is in addition a progesterone. This combination has been shown to be clinically effective in acne [10], and can reduce the SER by up to 75% [9]. In the combined oral contraceptives, the estrogen dose may be reduced by using 19-nortestosterone as the progesterone, but this compound has some androgenic activity and may indeed provoke or exacerbate acne [1]. Norethisterone, however, reduces circulating sex hormone binding levels to a lesser extent than norgestrel, and is used in the oral contraceptive Minovlar® (norethisterone 1 mg + ethinyl estradiol 50 μg). This combination has been shown to increase the SHBG [8], and reduce the SER [13].

The aim of this study was to determine by a randomized double-blind study whether cyproterone acetate adds significantly to the improvement of acne that occurs following treatment with estrogen, and to investigate the changes in androgen levels that occur during treatment with cyproterone acetate.

Methods

76 women with moderate to severe acne completed the trial (details see tab. 1). All acne medication except for the contraceptive pill was stopped for 6 weeks prior to therapy. All assessments were carried out at the mid-point of the cycle (between days 10—18 after the first day of menstrual bleeding). Patients had two base line examinations separated by one week before commencement of the trial, and then were assessed midway through the second, fourth and sixth cycle of treatment. At the initial visit they were stratified for severity using baseline total grades and randomly allocated to one of three treatment groups:

Group M (Minovlar®): Norethisterone acetate 1 mg and ethinyl estradiol 50 μg in a combined preparation taken daily from days 5—25 of cycle inclusive; plus placebo (to resemble CPA 50 mg tablets) taken daily from days 5—14 inclusive.

Group D (Diane®): Cyproterone acetate 2 mg and ethinyl estradiol 50 μg combined for days 5—25; plus placebo for days 5—14.

Group C (high dose CPA): Cyproterone acetate 50 mg for days 5—14; plus ethinyl estradiol 50 μg for days 5—25 as in the reversed sequential regimen of Hammerstein et al. [10].

Assessment

The severity of acne was graded according to the method of Burke & Cunliffe [4] by two observers separately for face, back and chest, and these grades were added together for a total grade. In addition the number of macules, papules, pustules, nodules and cysts on the face were recorded. Subjective changes were assessed using a visual analogue scale. Photographs were taken at each visit and these were graded by two observers.

The sebum excretion rate was measured by the method of Pochi and Strauss [11] with modifications [6]. Bacterial sampling for anaerobes (P. acnes) and aerobes (staphylococci and micrococci) was performed by the cup scrup tech-

Table 1 Details of age and weight of patients in each group

group	therapy	no. completing	age (years) mean and range	weight (kg) mean and range
M	Minovlar®	24	24.2 (18–36)	58.7 (58.3–59.2)
D	Diane®	26	24.2 (18–34)	58.6 (45.8–74.1)
C	High dose CPA	26	22.8 (16–30)	55.9 (43.5–80.0)

nique [17]. Numbers of colony forming bacteria were determined by plating out serial decimal dilutions onto tryptic soya agar recovery media, and expressed as the $\log_{10}$ colony-forming units per cm^2.

Blood was taken and the free and total testosterone and free and total dihydrotestosterone were measured by radioimmunoassay.

Results

There were no differences between the three treatment groups in respect to age or initial acne grading. There was significant difference in weight between those in group C and those in groups M and D ($p < 0.05$ Kruskal-Wallace test; tab. 1).

Clinical results

Both total (fig. 1) and facial (fig. 2) acne grades were improved in all groups following 6 months treatment, and significant reduction in grades had occurred after 2 months in groups D and C, and after 4 months in group M. At the end of the trial period both groups D and C had shown a significantly greater improvement than group M (Wilcoxon rank sum test), but group C, with a higher dose of cyproterone acetate than group D, showed a trend not reaching statisti-

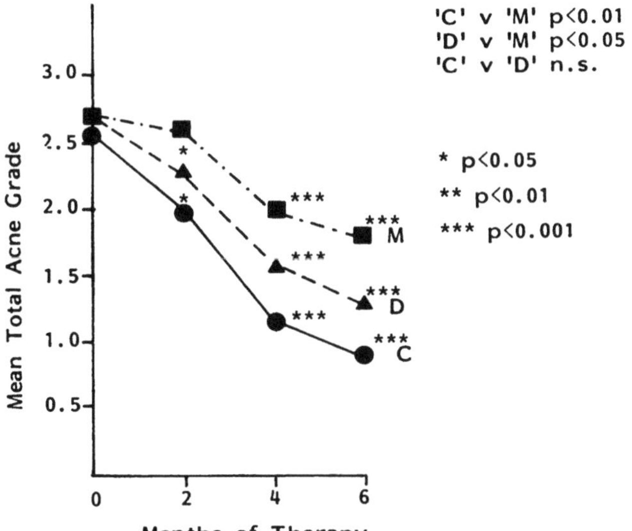

Fig. 1 Mean total acne grade at each visit during therapy with high dose cyproterone acetate (50 mg days 5—14) + ethinyl estradiol (50 µg days 5—25) (C); Diane (D); or Minovlar (M).

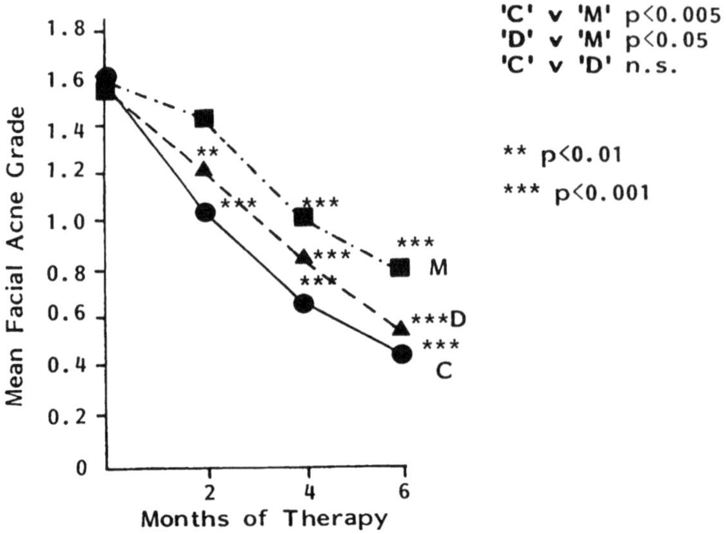

Fig. 2 Mean facial acne grade at each visit during therapy with high dose cyproterone acetate (50 mg days 5—14) + ethinyl estradiol (50 µg days 5—25) (C); Diane (D); or Minovlar (M).

Table 2

PAPULE COUNTS

Median ± SEM

TIME	C	D	M	Intergroup Stats
Baseline	26.5 ± 9.2	33.5 ± 6.8	29.5 ± 3.9	NS
2 Months	22.5 ± 4.7 (84.9%)	27.0 ± 6.6 (80.6%)	26.5 ± 4.2 (89.8%)	NS
4 Months	9.0 ± 2.4*** (34.0%)	13.5 ± 3.8** (40.3%)	24.0 ± 5.2 (81.4%)	D>C p<0.05 M>C p<0.01
6 Months	5.5 ± 2.6*** (20.8%)	15.0 ± 4.0** (44.8%)	19.5 ± 4.0 (66.1%)	D>C p<0.01 M>C p<0.01

* p<0.025
** p<0.005
*** p<0.001

cal significance towards greater improvement. These improvements were supported by the photographic assessments.

Individual lesion counts also demonstrated a reduction in numbers of papules (tab. 2). The number of papules was significantly reduced by 2 months in group C and by 4 months in group D. Group M by six months showed a trend only towards improvement. Reduction in pustules was more difficult to assess in view of fewer patients with large numbers of these lesions, but there was a statistically significant improvement in groups C and D by 2 months which did not occur in group M till 6 months (tab. 3). Subjective assessment by the patient using the visual analogue score demonstrated improvement in all groups (fig. 3), and in group C this was more marked than groups D or M which were comparable.

Investigations

a. Sebum excretion rate

The SER was markedly reduced in both groups D and C by 2 months with smaller reduction thereafter (fig. 4). Paralleling the clinical results, there was no

Table 3 **PUSTULE COUNTS**

Median values ± SEM Median

TIME	C	D	M	Intergroup Stats
Baseline	5.5 ± 3.2	4.5 ± 3.0	5.5 ± 2.4	NS
2 Months	2.0 ± 1.0*	2.5 ± 4.2*	6.0 ± 2.6	NS
4 Months	0 ± 0.7**	1.0 ± 2.4***	5.5 ± 2.5	C<D p<0.05 D<M p<0.05
6 Months	0 ± 0.6***	1.0 ± 1.3***	1.0 ± 1.1**	NS

* p<0.01
** p<0.005
*** p<0.001

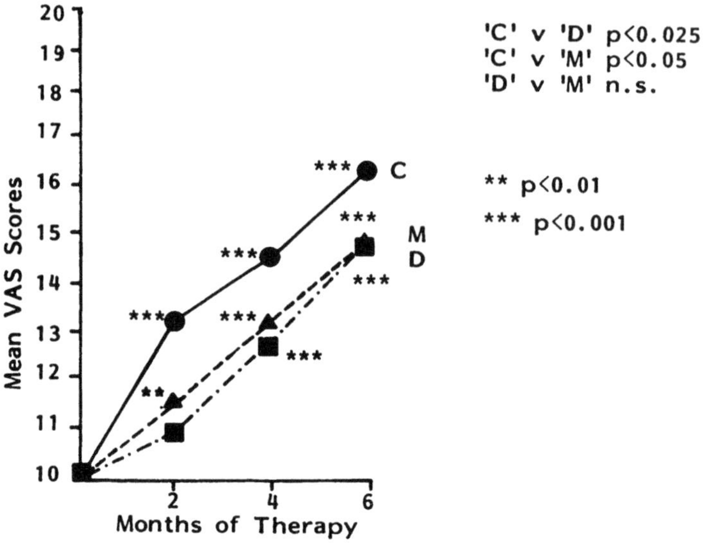

Fig. 3 Mean visual analogue score at each visit during therapy with high dose cyproterone acetate (50 mg days 5—14) + ethinyl estradiol (50 μg days 5—25) (C); Diane (D); or Minovlar (M).

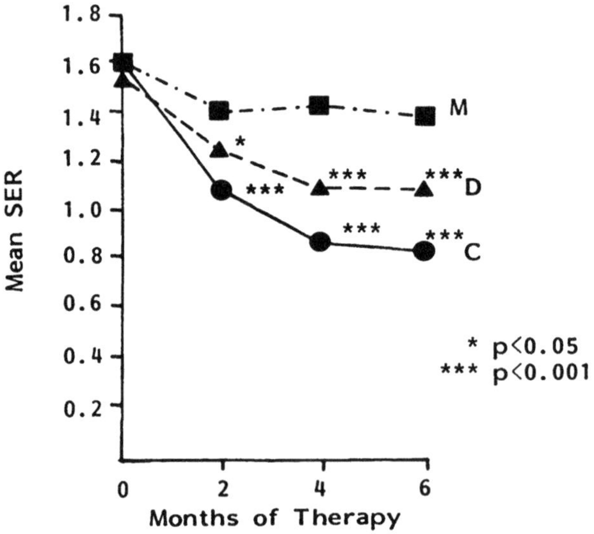

Fig. 4 Mean Sebum Excretion Rate at each visit during therapy with high dose cyproterone acetate (50 mg days 5—14) + ethinyl estradiol (50 μg days 5—25) (C); Diane (D); or Minovlar (M).

significant difference between groups D and C, although group C showed a definite trend towards a greater reduction in SER. There was no significant reduction in SER in group M by six months. Comparison of SER and clinical improvement in individual patients failed to demonstrate any significant correlation.

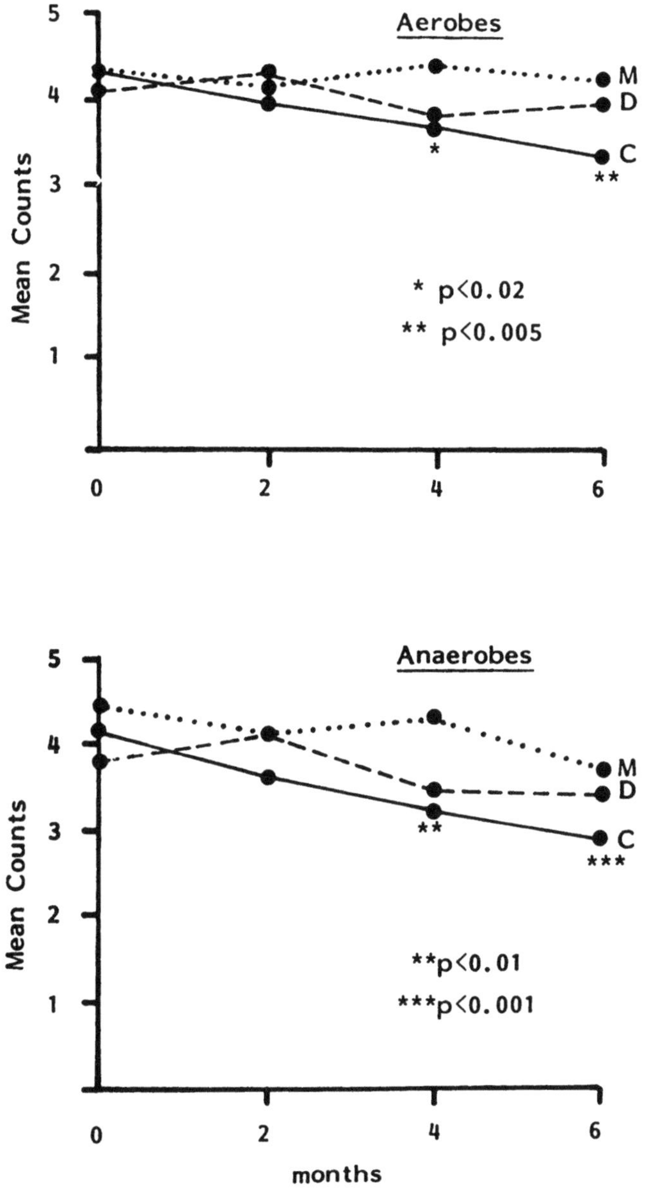

Fig. 5 Mean aerobic and anaerobic bacterial counts (log_{10} colony forming units per cm^2) during therapy with high dose cyproterone acetate (50 mg days 5—14) + ethinyl estradiol (50 μg days 5—25) (C); Diane (D); or Minovlar (M).

b. Bacterial counts

A significant reduction in anaerobic and aerobic bacterial counts (fig. 5) was noted in group C at 4 months, but not in either groups D or M. No correlation

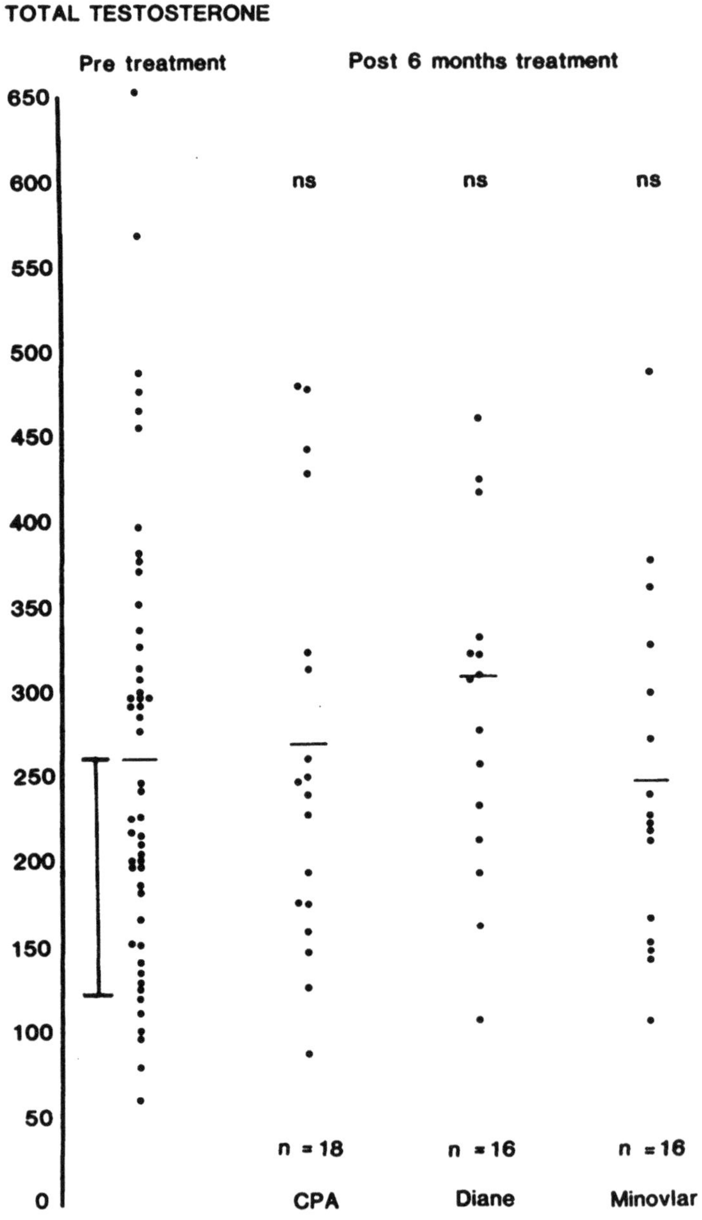

Fig. 6 Total testosterone levels pre-treatment and after 6 months therapy with high dose cyproterone acetate (50 mg days 5—14) + ethinyl estradiol (50 μg days 5—25) (C); Diane (D); of Minovlar (M) (normal range indicated by bar adjacent to vertical axis, mean value indicated by—).

between the bacterial counts and acne grade was found, but there was a significant relationship between $\log_{10}$ SER and decrease in the anaerobic bacterial count in group C.

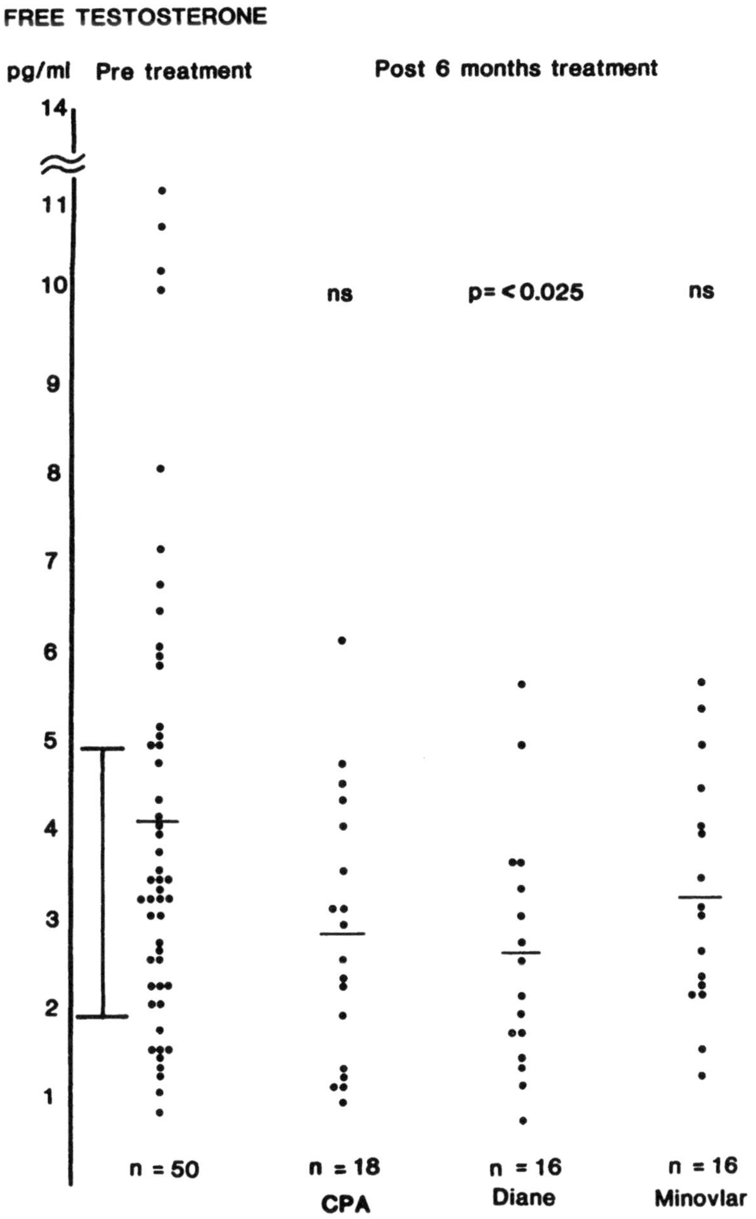

Fig. 7 Free testosterone levels pre-treatment and after 6 months therapy with high dose cyproterone acetate (50 mg days 5—14) + ethinyl estradiol (50 µg days 5—25) (C); Diane (D); of Minovlar (M) (normal range indicated by bar adjacent to vertical axis, mean value indicated by—).

c. Hormonal levels

No change in the total (fig. 6) or free testosterone (fig. 7) was observed following treatment in any of the three groups. There was no change in the wide range of total testosterone values from start to finish of the study. The range of the free testosterone levels (fig. 7) following treatment with both cyproterone ace-

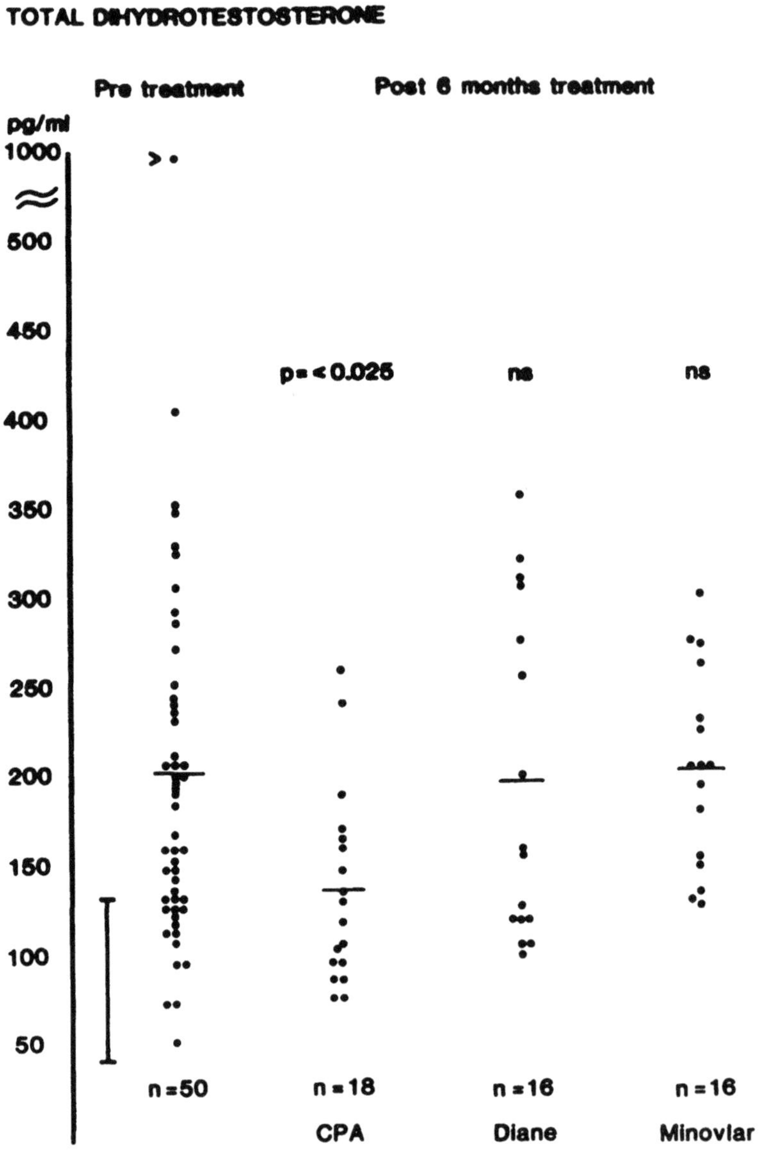

Fig. 8 Total dihydrotestosterone levels pre-treatment and after 6 months therapy with high dose cyproterone acetate (50 mg days 5—14) + ethinyl estradiol (50 µg days 5—25) (C); Diane (D); of Minovlar (M) (normal range indicated by bar adjacent to vertical axis, mean value indicated by—).

tate and estrogen alone was reduced with fewer very high values. However, because of the large variation in values, these were found not to be statistical significant from the initial values.

No statistical difference was seen in the total dihydrotestosterone levels (fig. 8) before and after treatment in any of the groups. In the group with high dose of cyproterone acetate (C), the levels of the free dihydrotestosterone (fig. 9) were significantly reduced ($p < 0.005$), but in groups M and D, no changes in the free dihydrotestosterone levels were observed.

Side effects

The major side effects encountered are listed in table 4. There were no differences in the number of patients with side effects or incidence of individual side

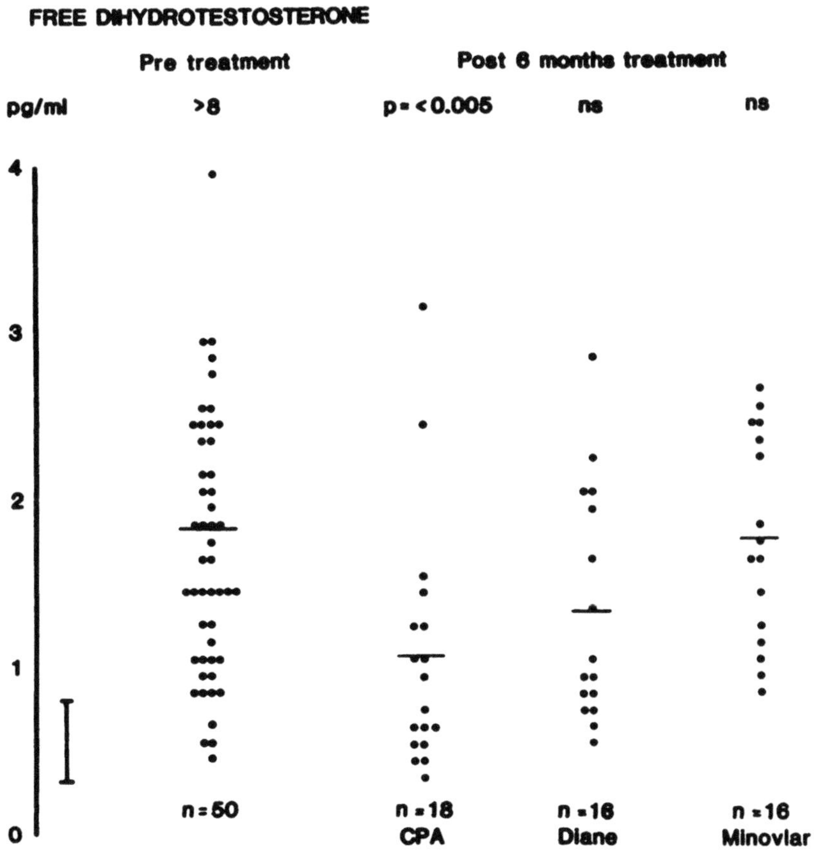

Fig. 9 Free dihydrotestosterone levels pre-treatment and after 6 months therapy with high dose cyproterone acetate (50 mg days 5—14) + ethinyl estradiol (50 µg days 5—25) (C); Diane (D); of Minovlar (M) (normal range indicated by bar adjacent to vertical axis, mean value indicated by—).

effects between the groups. 7/26, 8/26 and 6/26 of patients in groups D, C and M respectively reported no incidence of side effects. There was a highly significant tendency for side effects to be reported at the second month visit with a marked reduction later on.

Discussion

This trial demonstrates a significant clinical improvement in acne assessed objectively by clinical grading, photographic assessment, lesion counts and subjectively by visual analogue scores in all three treatment groups. A more rapid and effective response was seen with patients who were given cyproterone acetate, and no statistical difference was seen between the higher dose of 50 mg and the low 2 mg dose. The higher dose showed a consistent trend towards greater improvement in both clinical assessment and SER, and had a higher dose (100 mg) been used this may have reached statistical significance. Other investigators have suggested that after 12 months therapy there was little difference between Diane® and 100 mg of cyproterone acetate [2]. In the present study several patients with a poor response following the trial period showed good clinical results when given 100 mg of cyproterone acetate.

The rapid reduction in SER correlated with the use of cyproterone acetate and agreed with previous studies [7], and 50 µg of estrogen without cyproterone acetate in contradiction to other investigators [13] did not have any significant effect on SER. This would suggest that the cyproterone acetate is of prime importance in achieving clinical effectiveness.

Table 4 Side effects reported during the trial

Symptoms	treatment group		
	Minovlar®	Diane®	CPA
Tiredness/lassitude	5	1	5
Loss of libido	1	–	1
Headaches	5	4	7
Dizziness/giddiness	4	6	4
Breast soreness	5	6	6
Urgency of micturition	3	1	4
Depression	4	4	4
Nausea/vomiting	8	8	4
Abnormal uterine bleeding	3	3	5
Aching legs	1	–	3
Constipation	–	2	–
Abdominal pain	–	1	–
Benign breast tumour	–	1 (fibroadenosis)	–
Vaginal discharge	–	1 (cervical erosion)	–

No changes were seen in the total or free testosterone and total dihydrotestosterone levels before or after treatment. Only the highest dose of cyproterone acetate resulted in any reduction of the free dihydrotestosterone levels after treatment. However, all groups produced significant improvement in the acne, and this would suggest that the circulating hormone levels are unrelated to the severity of the acne. The effect of these hormones is therefore likely to be due to end organ sensitivity within the skin, rather than abnormally elevated levels in the blood.

Adverse effects were found in all treatment groups equally, and therefore were unlikely to be attributed to the anti-androgen itself. The side effects noted were similar to those found following treatment with the oral contraceptive with similar estrogen content [10].

Summary

Seventy-six patients with acne were randomly allocated to one of three treatment groups; Diane®, high dose cyproterone acetate (CPA) (50 mg) with ethinyl estradiol or Minovlar®. All treatment groups received the same dose of estrogen. Patients were assessed every two months for 6 months for the severity of acne by grading, lesion counts, and photography. In addition sebum excretion rate (SER), bacterial counts and hormonal levels (both total and free testosterone and dihydrotestosterone) were performed.

The results demonstrated clinical improvement in all three treatment groups, and a more rapid and effective response was seen in those groups treated with cyproterone acetate. These groups also demonstrated a reduction in SER, but no correlation was found between clinical improvement and reduction in SER in individual patients. No significant changes were found in the total and free testosterone and total dihydrotestosterone levels after treatment. A reduction in the level of free dihydrotestosterone was found only in those patients treated with high dose (50 mg) cyproterone acetate. We have demonstrated that the addition of cyproterone acetate to estrogen results in a more effective therapeutic result in the treatment of acne, and that acne is related to the effect of the testosterones in the skin, rather than to raised circulating hormones.

References

[1] Barranco, V. P., D. D. Jones: Effect of oral contraceptives on acne. Southern Medical Journal **67** (1974) 703.

[2] Breckwoldt, M., R. Trolp, W. Braendle et al.: Anti-androgen oral contraceptives. In: Haspels, A. A., C. R. Kay (eds.): International Symposium on Hormonal Contraception, p. 81. Excerpta Medica Intern. Congress Series 441, Amsterdam 1978.

[3] Bruckovsky, N.: Molecular action of androgens and antiandrogens. In: Hammerstein, J., L. Lachnit-Fixson, F. Neumann et al. (eds.): Androgenization in Women, p. 11. Exerpta Medica, Amsterdam 1980.
[4] Burke, B. M., W. J. Cunliffe: The assessment of acne vulgaris—the Leeds technique. British Journal of Dermatology **111** (1984) 83.
[5] Burton, J. L., S. Shuster: The relationship between seborrhoea and acne vulgaris. British Journal of Dermatology **84** (1971) 600.
[6] Cunliffe, W. J., S. M. Williams, S. G. Tan: Sebum excretion rate investigations. British Journal of Dermatology **93** (1975) 347.
[7] Ebling, F. J., A. K. Thomas, I. D. Cooke et al.: Effect of cyproterone acetate on hair growth, sebaceous excretion and endocrine parameters in a hirsute subject. British Journal of Dermatology **97** (1977) 371.
[8] El Makhazangy, M. N., V. Wynn, D. M. Lawrence: Sex hormone binding globulin capacity as an index of oestrogenicity or androgenicity in women on oral contraceptive steroids. Clinical Endocrinology **10** (1979) 39.
[9] Fanta, D., M. M. Muller: Effect of cyproterone acetate on skin surface lipids. Acta Dermato-venereologica **58** (1978) 85.
[10] Hammerstein, J., J. Meckies, I. Leo-Rossberg et al.: The use of cyproterone acetate in the treatment of acne, hirsutism and virilism. Journal of Steroid Biochemistry **6** (1975) 827.
[11] Pochi, P. E., J. S. Strauss: The quantitative gravimetric determination of sebum production. Journal of Investigative Dermatology **36** (1961) 293.
[12] Pochi, P. E., J. S. Strauss: Sebaceous gland suppression with ethinyl estradiol and diethylstilbestrol. Archives of Dermatology **108** (1973) 210.
[13] Pye, R. J., G. Meyrick, M. J. Pye et al.: Effect of oral contraceptives on sebum excretion rate. British Medical Journal **1** (1977) 1581.
[14] Schleusener, A., F. Neumann: Antiandrogens — scientific and experimental background. In: Orfanos, C. E., W. Montagna, G. Stuttgen (eds.): Hair Research, p. 322. Springer-Verlag, Berlin 1981.
[15] Strauss, J. S., A. M. Kligman, P. E. Pochi: The effect of androgens and estrogens on human sebaceous glands. Journal of Investigative Dermatology **39** (1962) 139.
[16] Shuster, S., M. F. Cooper, D. McGibbon et al.: Epidermal lipid synthesis in acne. British Journal of Dermatology **103** (1980) 127.
[17] Williamson, P., A. M. Kligman: A new method for the quantitative investigation of cutaneous bacteria. Journal of Investigative Dermatology **45** (1965) 498.

IV Special aspects

Clinical assessment of two antiandrogen treatments, cyproterone acetate combined with ethinyl estradiol and spironolactone in hirsutism

R. Rubens, A. Vermeulen

Introduction

Cyproterone acetate (CPA) combined with ethinyl estradiol (EE_2) has been used for the treatment of hirsutism [12]. Recently, spironolactone has also been introduced as an antiandrogen for the treatment of hirsutism. Reports concerning its efficacity have been published mainly by North American and Italian groups [1]. Few comparisons between these two antiandrogen treatments based on objective criteria have so far been reported. We therefore compared the results of both treatment schedules in hirsute women.

Patients and methods

Patients consulting for dysfunctional hirsutism were selected for treatment. Hirsutism was scored according to the Ferriman and Gallwey scoring system by two physicians; this was repeated after 3, 6, and 12 months of treatment. Before treatment each patient was investigated to exclude Cushing syndrome, congenital hyperplasia, and ovarian or adrenal tumors. The remaining patients were considered to have dysfunctional hirsutism. Patients having a dominantly ovarian hirsutism (assessed by a 5-day Dexamethasone test) were treated with cyproterone acetate 50 mg/day from the 5th to the 16th day of the cycle. This was combined with ethinyl estradiol 50 μg from the 5th to the 26th day of the cycle. Patients having an increased 5α reductase (i. e., only increased 5α diol) received treatment with spironolactone. Clinical parameters were, however, similar.

Spironolactone was administered in a 100 mg dose from the 5th to the 26th day of the cycle. Statistical analysis was performed using the paired Wilcoxon or the Mann-Whitney test. For qualitative measurements a simple chi-square test was used.

Results

In table 1 the clinical parameters of the two groups of patients are presented. Antropometric measurements were similar in both groups. The only noticeable difference between both groups was the menstrual status: oligomenorrhea was more frequent in the cyproterone acetate/ethinyl estradiol group; regular menstrual cycles were more frequent in the spironolactone group. Results of treatment are reported in figure 1. As can be seen, both treatment schedules induced a significant improvement of the Ferriman and Gallwey score; after three months of treatment improvement was already statistically significant. In the

Table 1 Clinical parameters

		Treatment	
		Spiro	CPA + EE 2
N		23	35
Age (years)		24 ± 7	23 ± 7
Weight (kg)		67 ± 13	61 ± 14
Height (m.)		1.65 ± 0.06	1.63 ± 0.06
BMI		24 ± 5	23 ± 5
Menstrual	Rg	13	11
status (*)	Oligo	10	24

(*) chi-square = 0.1

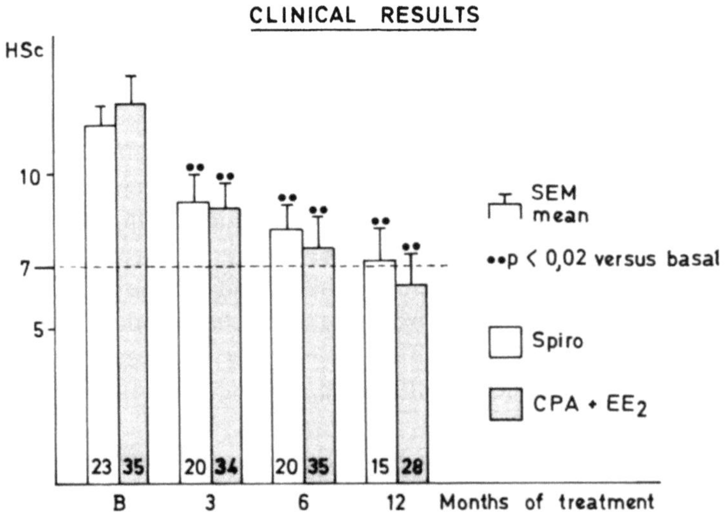

Fig. 1 Clinical assessment of two antiandrogen treatments, cyproterone acetate combined with ethinyl estradiol and spironolactone in hirsutism

cyproterone acetate/ethinyl estradiol group the mean Ferriman and Gallwey score after 12 months of treatment was within the limits for the normal population. Spironolactone, on the other hand, produced slightly less impressive results.

As to individual results, a much higher percentage of patients showed improvement or even normalization after cyproterone acetate/ethinyl estradiol treatment than after spironolactone (tab. 2). The total failure rate with spironolactone, 35% (tab. 4), is higher than the failure rate with cyproterone acetate/ethinyl estradiol, 20% (tab. 3).

Concerning side-effects, cyproterone acetate/ethinyl estradiol patients complained of tiredness upon specific questioning (n = 15) and sometimes had slight breast tenderness (n = 5). There were no drop-outs in this group.

Spironolactone caused polymenorrhea at the beginning of the treatment in the majority of patients (n = 14). The polymenorrhea disappeared, however, after 3 or 6 months in most patients. Breast tenderness was sometimes present in some patients (n = 2) but there was no complaint about tiredness. The drop out rate was 3/23 patients : one moved, one wished contraception, and the third refused further treatment after 3 months of treatment.

Table 2 Influence of treatment (12 months) on hirsutism

	Total treated	Cured	Improved
CPA + EE2	35	23	+ 5 = 28
Spiro	23	8(*)	+ 4 = 12(*)

Cured: F & G-score < 7 at 6 or 12 months
Improved: decrease of F & G-score by 25% at 6 or 12 months
(*): $P < 0.05$

Table 3 Individual response to cyproterone acetate: FERRIMAN-GALLWEY-score before and during treatment

N = 35	
– Total failure: F & G-score at 12 months = basal score:	7 = 20%
– Improved: F & G-score at 6 or 12 months < 75% basal score:	5 = 14%
– Normalized: F & G-score after 12 months ≤ 7:	23 = 66%

Table 4 Individual response to spironolactone

N = 23	
Insufficient data:	3 = 13%
Total failure:	8 = 35%
Improved:	4 = 17%
Normalized:	8 = 35%

Discussion

Both antiandrogen treatments have a beneficial effect upon hirsutism; the effect of cyproterone acetate/ethinyl estradiol is, however, more consistent and more pronounced. This is explained by the three effects of this combination: (1) antiandrogenicity strictu sensu; (2) progestative effect on the pituitary which results in lowering of ovarian androgen secretion [5]; (3) increase of TeBG and thus decrease of free 17β ol androgens available to the tissues.

The antiandrogenic effect of cyproterone acetate is due to three main mechanisms:

(1) It blocks the testosterone receptor [2, 9].

(2) It inhibits 5α reductase activity in the skin of hirsute patients treated concurrently with ethinyl estradiol [12]. Whether this is a direct effect of cyproterone acetate or this is due to the lowering of the androgens by the combination remains a matter of controversy. Mowszowicz et al. [10] reported an increased 5α diol glucuronide excretion under cyproterone acetate and estrogen treatment. We, however, observed a decreased 5α diol in plasma [12]. Cyproterone acetate induces hepatic enzymes and increases the smooth endoplasmatic reticulum in rat hepatocytes [6] as well as glucuronide formation [11]. The interpretation of 5α diol glucuronide measurements is difficult.

(3) Finally, cyproterone acetate combined with estrogens causes an increase in the metabolic clearance rate of androgens [10] and thus a decrease in circulating androgens.

The effect of spironolactone is also based on a spectrum of biological effects: spironolactone is an antiandrogen too: it binds to the androgen receptor in vitro [15]. It also reduces 5α reductase activity [14]. It does not increase TeBG concentration, but rather decreases it so that the androgens are more available to the target tissues [7]. Spironolactone, in a high dose ($>$ 100 mg/day), is also a weak progestagen [13]. This progestagen effect does not decrease the gonadotrophin levels, however, but causes mid-cycle bleedings.

Spironolactone also interferes with the microsomal P-450 content. It inhibits 17β hydroxylase and 17—20 desmolase activity in the rodent and dog adrenal [8]. This effect was suggested as the cause of the decrease of the androgens observed in some studies [3, 4]. Later reports claimed this effect to be less consistent [4]. Furthermore, searches for an explanation of the non-effectiveness in certain patients reported in these latter reports made it evident that certain previously described effects were due to patient selection [3]. Detailed results of spironolactone treatment have seldom been reported. Some authors advocate combination with an oral contraceptive [1, 15] to increase effectiveness.

The secondary effects of spironolactone are less well accepted by the patients than those of cyproterone acetate. The major complaint is polymenorrhea which is probably due to the slight progestagenic effect of spironolactone

[13]. One patient showed a slight increase of transaminases (toxic hepatitis?).

The main advantage of spironolactone treatment seems to be the persistence of ovarian ovulatory activity during treatment preserving and even sometimes restoring fertility. We advise our patients to stop treatment when pregnancy has occurred, as the effects of this weak antiandrogen during pregnancy have not been thoroughly tested in the dosage as used here. The financial burden of both treatment schedules is similar, approximatly 10 Dollars a month.

In summary, we conclude that both antiandrogens are effective in the treatment of hirsutism. The overall efficiency of cyproterone acetate is, however, better than that of spironolactone. Both drugs are well tolerated, but spironolactone can cause troublesome polymenorrhea.

References

[1] Biffignandi, P., C. Massuchetti, G. M. Molinatti: Female hirsutism: Pathophysiological considerations and therapeutic implications. Endocrin. Reviews **5** (1984) 498—513.

[2] Bruchovsky, N.: Molecular actions of androgens and anti-androgens. In: Hammerstein et al. (eds.): Androgenisation in women, pp. 7—21. Excerpta Medica Congress Series, N° 493, 1980.

[3] Cumming, D. C., J. C. Yang, R. W. Rebar et al.: Treatment of hirsutism with spironolactone. JAMA **247** (1982) 1295—1298.

[4] Dorrington-Ward, P., A. C. E. McCartney, S. Holland et al.: The effect of spironolactone on hirsutism and female androgen metabolism. Clin. Endocr. **23** (1985) 161—167.

[5] Frey, H., A. Aakvaag: The treatment of essential hirsutism in women with cyproterone acetate and ethinyl oestradiol. Acta Obstet. Gynec. Scand. **60** (1981) 295—300.

[6] Garg, B., J. Diascheck, K. Kovacs: A comparative ultrastructural study on drug-induced proliferation of smooth endoplasmatic reticulum in hepatocytes. Tokohu. J. exp. Med. **104** (1971) 205—214.

[7] Manni, A., W. M. Pardridge, W. Cefalu et al.: Bioavailability of albumin-bound testosterone. J. clin. Endocrin. Metab. **61** (1985) 705—710.

[8] Menard, R. H., T. M. Guenther, H. Kon et al.: Studies on the destruction of adrenal and testicular cytochrome P-450 by spironolactone. J. biol. Chem. **254** (1979) 1726—1731.

[9] Mowszowicz, I., M. Rahi, F. Wright et al.: Androgen receptors in human skin cytosol. J. clin. Endocrin. Metab. **52** (1981) 338—344.

[10] Mowszowicz, I., F. Wright, M. Vincencs et al.: Androgen metabolism in hirsute patients treated with cyproterone acetate. J. Steroid. Biochem. **20** (1984) 757—761.

[11] Neumann, F., H. Steibeck: Antiandrogens. In: Eickler, O. et al. (eds.): Handbook of experimental pharmacology, pp. 428—434. Springer Verlag, Berlin. Part II, 1974.

[12] Rubens, R.: Androgen levels during cyproterone acetate and ethinyl oestradiol treatment of hirsutism. Clin. Endocrin. **20** (1984) 313—325.
[13] Schane, H. P., G. O. Potts: Oral progestagenic activity of spironolactone. J. clin. Endocrin. Metab. **47** (1978) 691—694.
[14] Serafini, P. C., J. Catalino, R. A. Lobo: The effect of spironolactone on genital skin 5 alpha-reductase activity. J. Steroid. Biochem. **23** (1985) 191—194.
[15] Tremblay, R. R.: Treatment of hirsutism with spironolactone. Clin. Endocrin. Metab. **15** (1986) 363—371.

Treatment of severe androgenization symptoms with Diane® and intramuscularly applied cyproterone acetate (Androcur® Depot)

E. Kaiser

Introduction

Today, various methods to treat androgen-induced endocrinopathy are available. The choice of therapy depends on the objective of the treatment: regression of virilism not due to a tumor, normalization of ovarian function or both. In addition, the therapy form is affected decisively by the personal wishes of the patient [8].

Experience with the anti-androgenic progestagens cyproterone acetate and chlormadinone acetate in the treatment of androgenization symptoms in women has now been available for more than 20 years [1, 14].

Nowadays, application of hormonal contraceptives with progestagens and ethinyl estradiol or mestranol is the treatment of choice for women with slight to moderately severe acne, slight to moderately severe hirsutism and androgenetic alopecia provided there is no present desire for children [5].

Especially in the severe form of androgenization but even in moderately severe forms the regression of symptoms has a protracted onset or the results are inadequate [12], so that it is necessary to raise the dose of antiandrogens in order to achieve the desired results. Cyproterone acetate (CPA) is appropriate either in the form of Androcur® 10 mg or Androcur® 50 mg depending on the severity of the androgenetic symptoms. It must be born in mind that according to Hammerstein and Cupceancu [4], cyproterone acetate has a certain depot character, so that its additional application must be carried out in a reversed cyclic manner in order to avoid delayed onset of withdrawal bleeding.

Cyproterone acetate is also available as Androcur® Depot, which is injected intramuscularly. As shown by investigations in patients with prostate carcinoma [10] and sexual deviations [11], a single injection of 300 mg of the substance in an oily solution has a clinical effect which corresponds to that of 100 mg oral cyproterone acetate daily. First investigations with the parenteral applicable cyproterone acetate depot preparation for the treatment of women with symptoms of androgenization were carried out by Moltz et al. [13]. Despite the smaller amount of cyproterone acetate per unit of time, he found a certain clinical superiority over oral therapy. Side effects corresponded to the high-dose standard oral treatment in nature and frequency.

The present investigation was carried out in women with severe androgenization symptoms such as very severe acne and/or pronounced hirsutism which were not due to tumors. The objective of the study was to examine whether comparable clinical results can be attained with the intramuscular administration form of cyproterone acetate together with the oral antiovulatory combination preparation Diane® which are comparable to those obtained with the oral reverse sequential scheme with which we have many years of experience [6, 7].

The therapeutic effects on the androgenization symptoms were registered together with tolerance and hormone parameters.

Materials and methods

Forty otherwise healthy women with exceedingly severe androgenization manifestations not due to tumors were included in the study.

The average age was 31.5 years (R: 16—57); height, 156.5 cm (R: 152—172); and body weight, 61.4 kg (R: 45—100).

The treatment was carried out with Androcur® Depot (300 mg cyproterone acetate in oily solution) and Diane® (2 mg cyproterone acetate and 0.05 mg ethinyl estradiol) (fig. 1).

On the first day of treatment of each therapy cycle, one ampoule of Androcur® Depot was applied intramuscularly; on the seventh day, patients started taking Diane® from the calender pack and then took one dragee daily for 21 days; after a pause of seven days, the treatment was continued in accordance with the same scheme over a further 11 treatment cycles.

The results of monthly checks by the same investigator were recorded on a progress sheet in which the degrees of severity of the androgenization symptoms were noted.

300 mg cyproterone acetate (CPA) in oily solution i. m. (= 1 ampoule SH 8.0714 300 mg = Androcur® Depot)
in combination with
1 tablet at 2 mg CPA + 0.05 mg Ethinyl estradiol per day for 21 days (= SH B 209 AB = Diane®)
7-day interval

Fig. 1 Application in the study

The following biochemical parameters were determined in the blood serum before the beginning of treatment and after 6 and 12 treatment cycles: fasting glucose, protein, alkaline phosphatase, GOT, GPT, LAP, gamma-GT, cholesterol, triglycerides, LDL and HDL. The hormone parameters testosterone, dehydroepiandrosterone sulfate, androstenedione, SHBG and prolactin were also measured.

In addition, the internal structure of the liver was evaluated in each patient at the beginning of treatment and after 12 treatment cycles, using ultrasonography with the rapid B imaging technique. A Kretz Combison 150 sector scanner (axial resolution 0.8 mm, lateral resolution 1.2 mm, frequency 3.0 MHz) was used for the investigations.

Results

Improvement of androgenization symptoms was mixed. Acne always improved, but disorders of hair pattern often did not respond satisfactorily. Facial hair in the form of beard growth was especially refractory.

Intermenstrual bleeding or anomalies of cycle tempo were slight and rare and did not give rise to any problems for the patients.

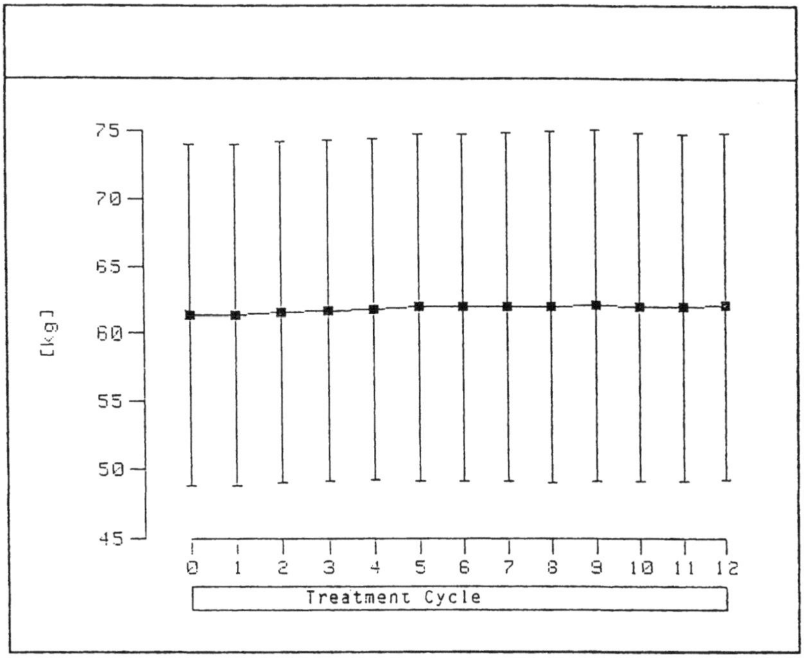

Fig. 2 Mean and standard deviations of body weight under treatment

Most patients could regulate the initial increase in weight of 1 kg to 2 kg by dietetic measures. Since a similarly large number of patients showed a decrease in weight under the treatment weight gain is not an automatic tendency under the treatment (fig. 2). Blood pressure remained constant during the whole observation period (fig. 3).

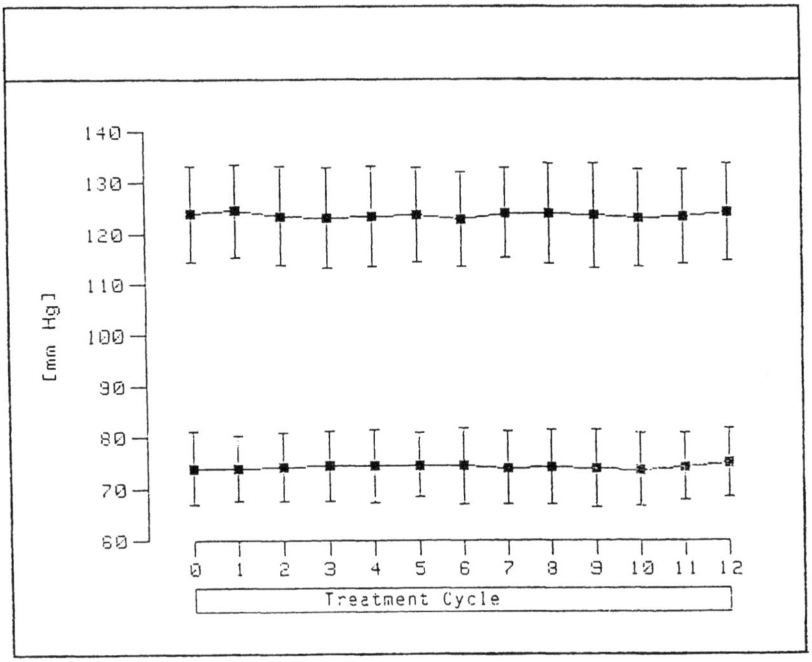

Fig. 3 Mean and standard deviations of blood pressure under treatment

Of the biochemical parameters of the glucose, liver (figs. 4—7) and lipid (figs. 8—11) metabolism, individual values were occasionally found to be outside the normal range both before the beginning of treatment and under treatment. Corresponding clinical symptoms were not present, and control measurements in the further course of treatment showed normalization. In no case was it necessary to interrupt therapy.

The hormone parameters of androgen metabolism were raised before the beginning of treatment in the majority of cases, but not in all patients. They were never in a range (testosterone more than 1.5 ng/ml, DHEA-S more than 7000 ng/ml) which suggested a tumor-induced hirsutism. In the course of treatment, there was a marked decrease of testosterone in 11 cases, of DHEA-S in 16 cases and of androstenedione in 22 cases. In the remaining patients, these hormone levels remained unchanged. Indeed, there was occasionally a slight rise.

The examinations of the internal structure of the liver by means of ultrasonography revealed a slight fatty degeneration of the parenchyma in 4 cases. In 3

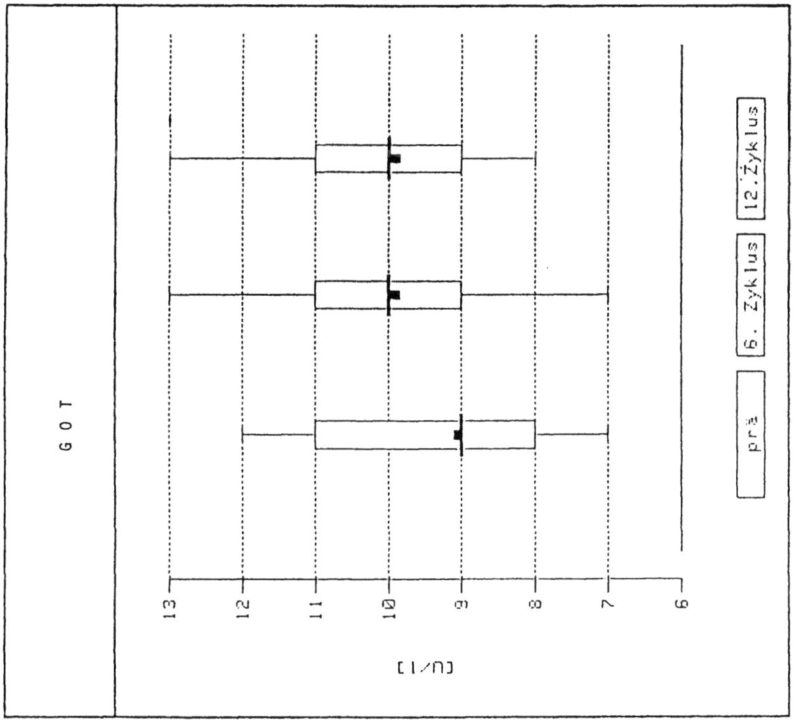
G O T
[U/l]
13
12
11
10
9
8
7
6
prä
6. Zyklus
12. Zyklus

Fig. 4

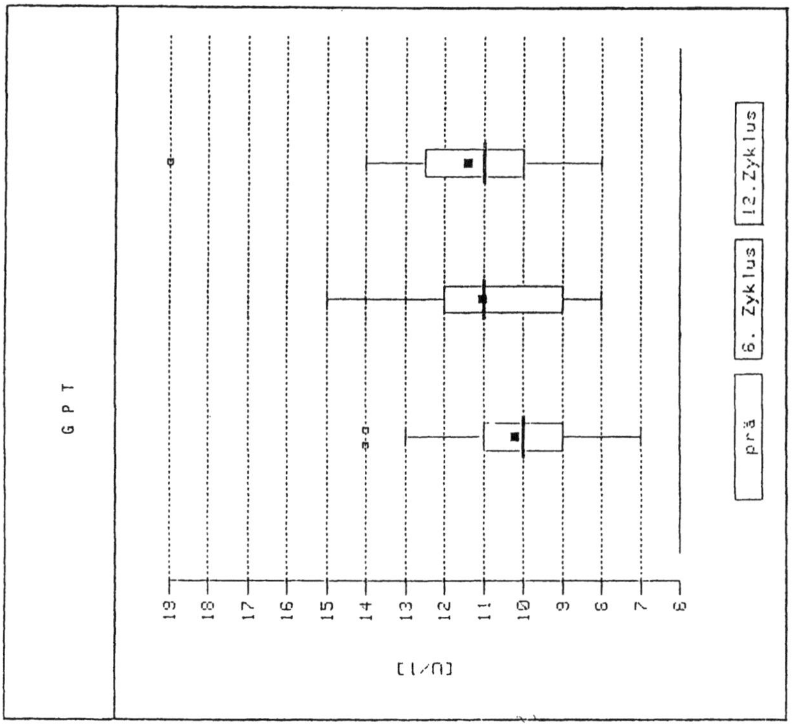
G P T
[U/l]
19
18
17
16
15
14
13
12
11
10
9
8
7
6
prä
6. Zyklus
12. Zyklus

Fig. 5

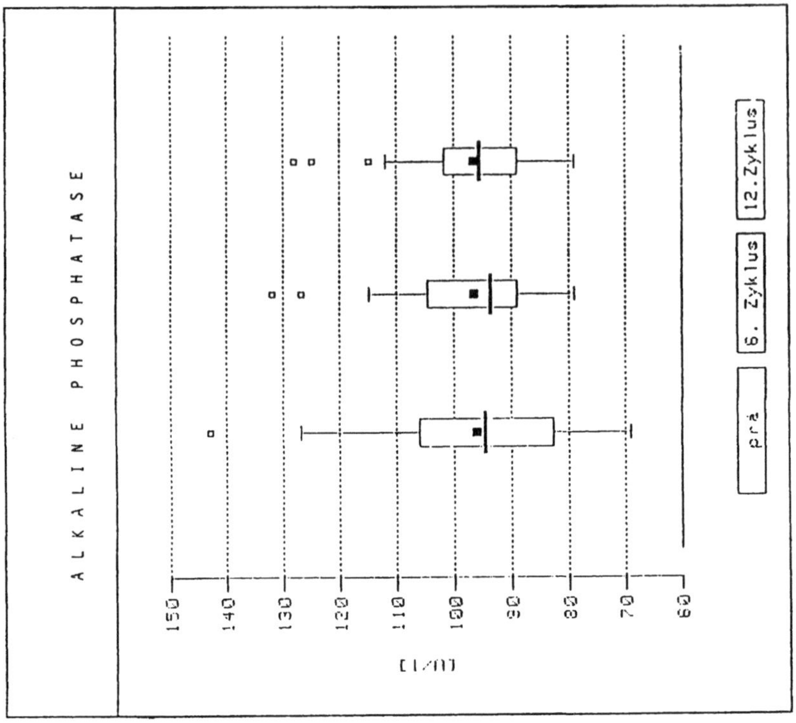
ALKALINE PHOSPHATASE
[U/l]
150
140
130
120
110
100
90
80
70
60
prä
6. Zyklus
12. Zyklus

Fig. 6

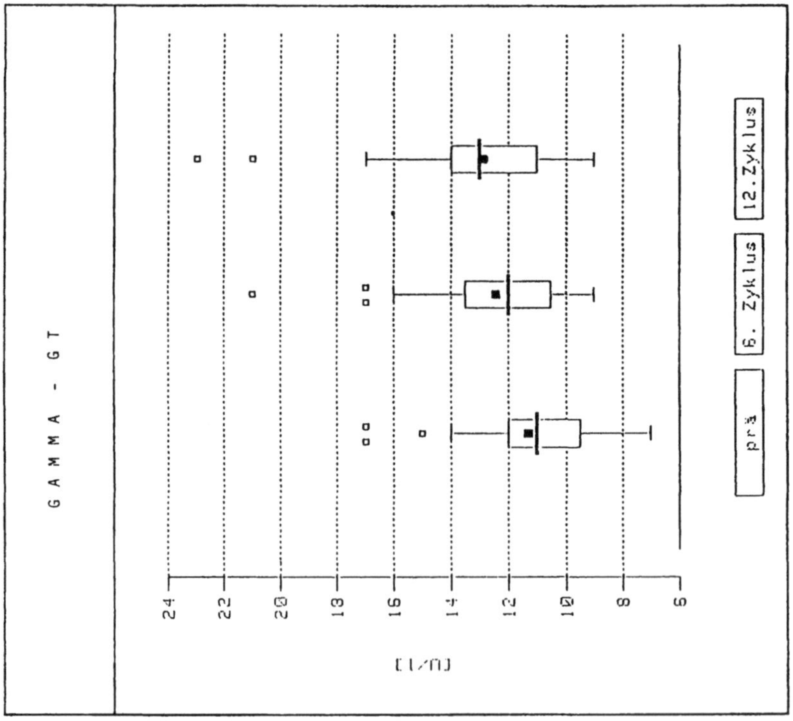
GAMMA - GT
[U/l]
24
22
20
18
16
14
12
10
8
6
prä
6. Zyklus
12. Zyklus

Fig. 7

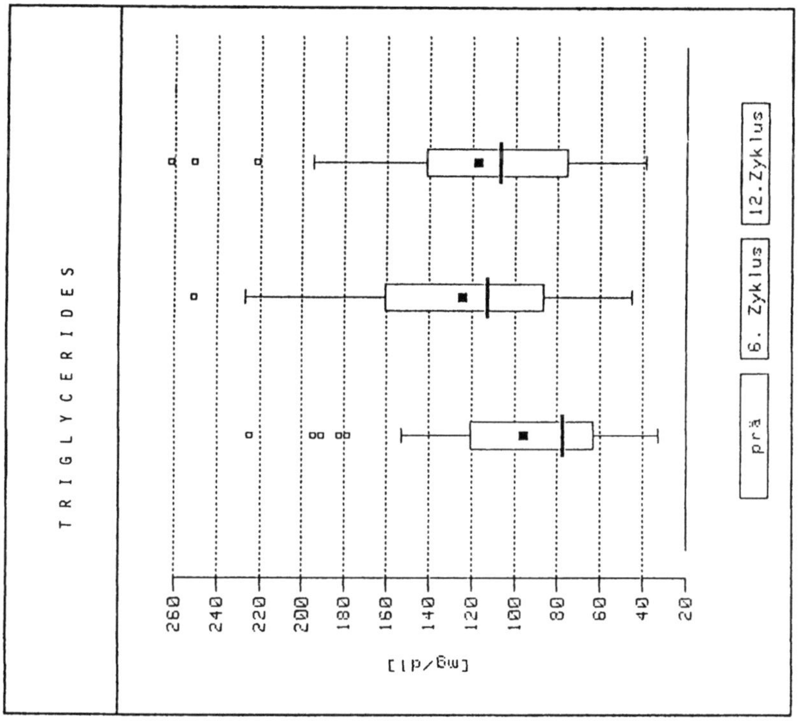
T R I G L Y C E R I D E S
[mg/dl]
260
240
220
200
180
160
140
120
100
80
60
40
20
prä
6. Zyklus
12.Zyklus

Fig. 8

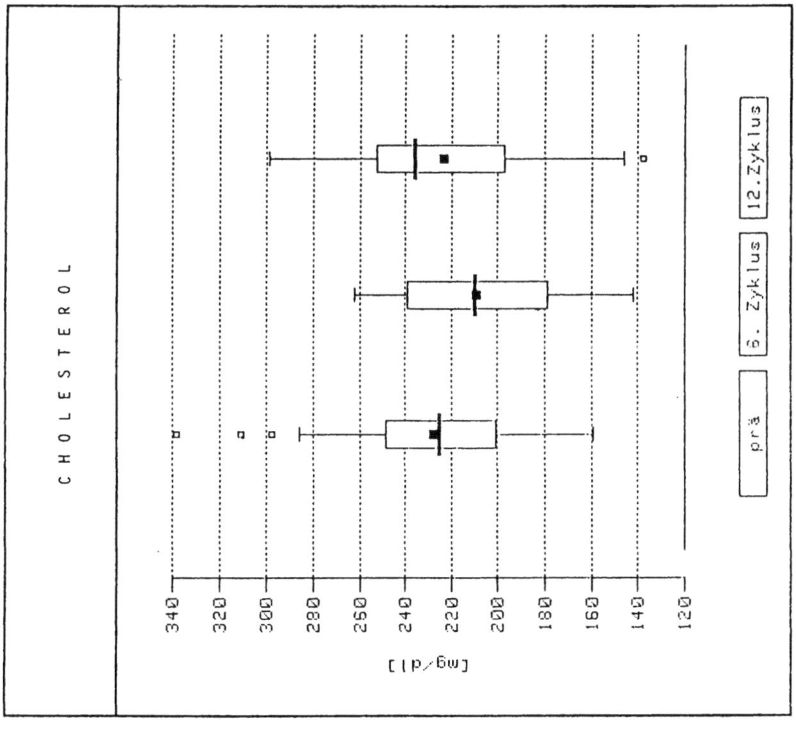
C H O L E S T E R O L
[mg/dl]
340
320
300
280
260
240
220
200
180
160
140
120
prä
6. Zyklus
12.Zyklus

Fig. 9

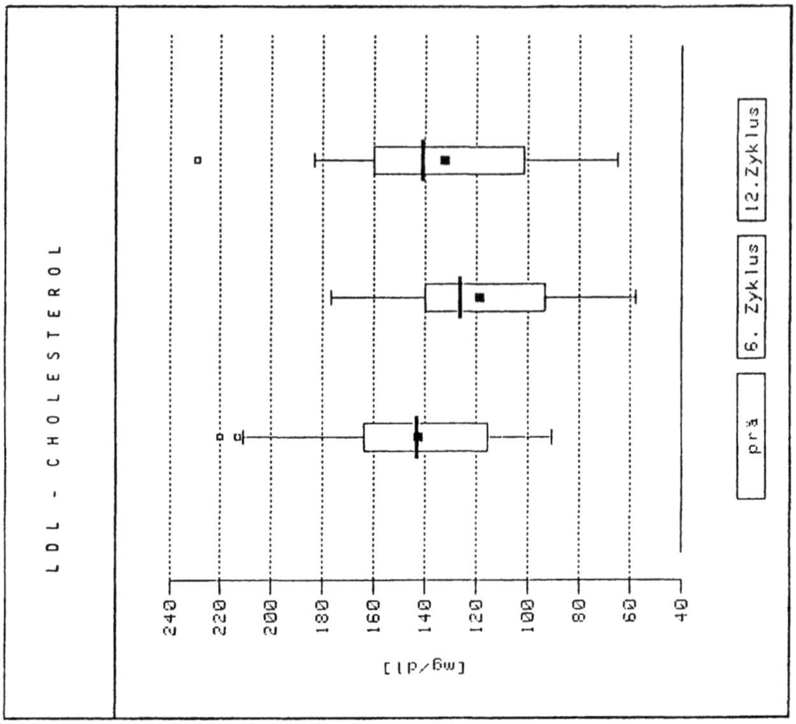
L D L - C H O L E S T E R O L
[mg/dl]
240
220
200
180
160
140
120
100
80
60
40
prä
6. Zyklus
12. Zyklus

Fig. 10

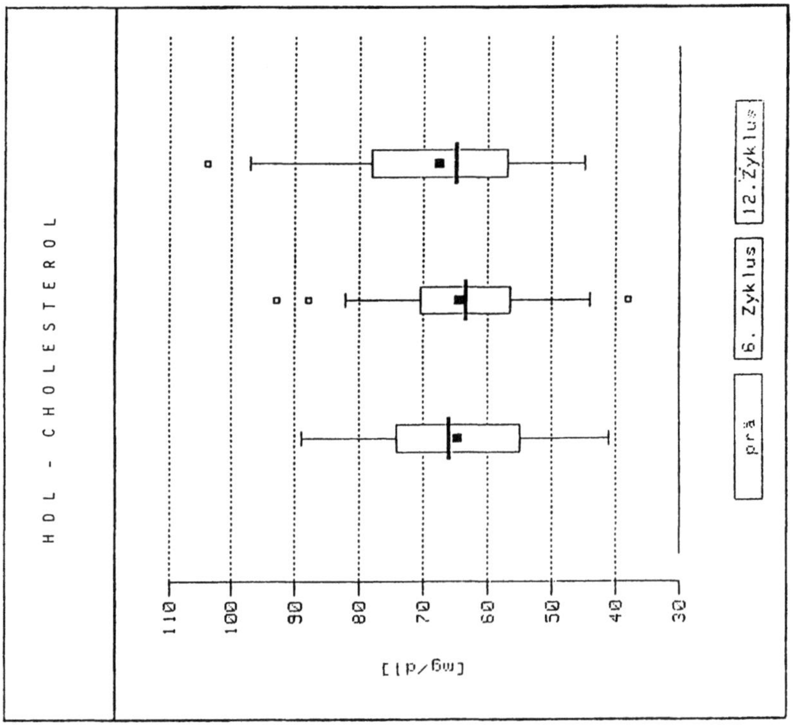
H D L - C H O L E S T E R O L
[mg/dl]
110
100
90
80
70
60
50
40
30
prä
6. Zyklus
12. Zyklus

Fig. 11

of these patients, obesity in connection with the hormone therapy may have played a role. Other possible causes such as taking drugs or latent or manifest diabetes could not be established in any of these cases. Since the alterations were slight, no alteration of the therapeutic concept was made. Follow-up examinations are foreseen. Two further patients already showed a slight fatty degeneration of the parenchyma before the beginning of treatment. No deterioration in the finding was detected at the check-up after 12 months of treatment.

Discussion

Under the treatment with Androcur® Depot (300 mg CPA i. m.) + Diane® in 40 women with pronounced androgenization symptoms, the androgen values showed a tendency to normalize. However, an increase was occasionally also detected, in particular an increase of dehydroepiandrosterone sulfate (figs 12,

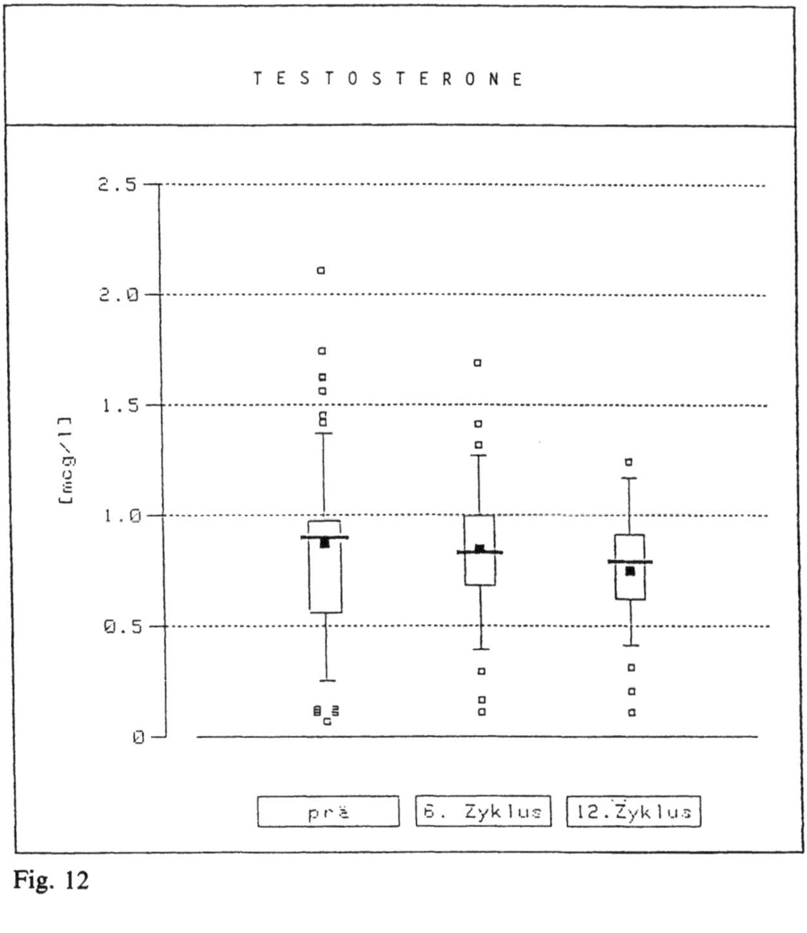

Fig. 12

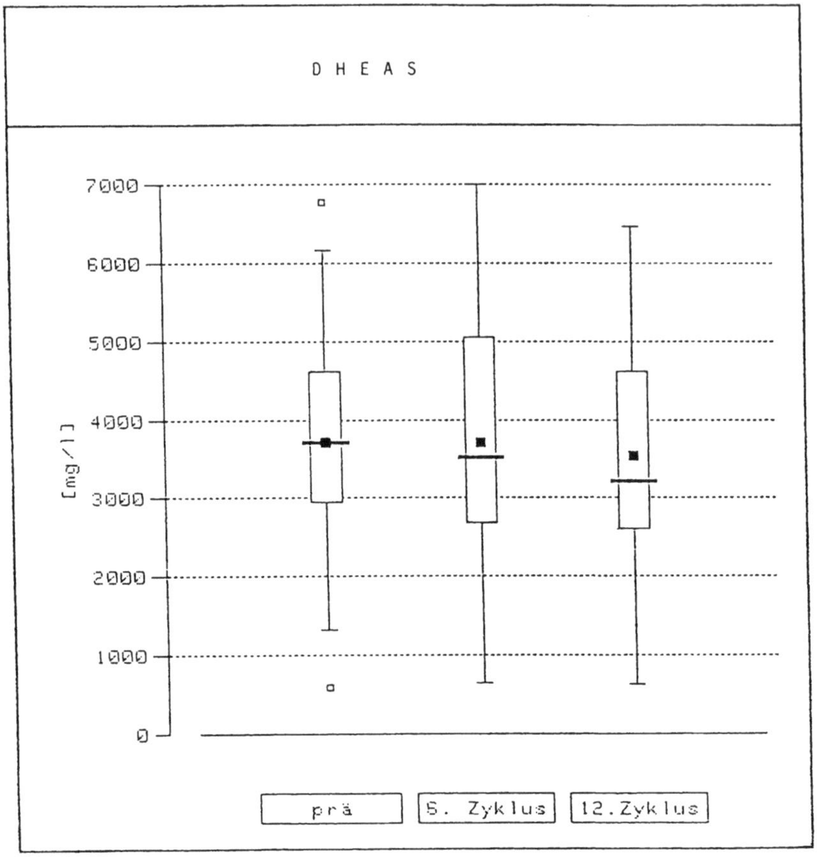

Fig. 13

13). It should be noted here that the initial values were not raised above normal in some of the patients. The inclusion of patients in the study was based on the clinical criterion of pronounced hirsutism irrespective of the laboratory parameters of androgen metabolism. The hormone curves were also not used to evaluate the result of therapy, since it has been shown that the clinical course and laboratory parameters do not necessarily conform in all cases [5, 12]. This is probably connected with the fact that raised androgen levels are not always present in hirsutism. Even in pronounced cases, a raised sensitivity of the androgenic target organs may be the decisive pathogenetic factor [16].

The result of therapy was appraised subjectively on the basis of the evaluation of the external appearance, i. e. the alteration in the disturbed hair pattern. The results of treatment correspond to those seen under the reverse sequential scheme according to Hammerstein [4] in which 1000 mg cyproterone acetate/cycle were administered orally (300 mg cyproterone acetate/cycle i. m. in this study).

The side effects appear to be fewer. We saw fewer pronounced cases of mastodynia and in contrast to Moltz et al. [13], we did not see any case of galactorrhea. The prolactin levels rose (fig. 14) as described by Flückiger et al. [2] under estrogens alone and by Moltz et al. [12] as well as by Frölich et al. [3] under cyproterone acetate in combination with estrogens. However, they usually remained within the normal range.

With regard to a possible influence of high-dose steroid therapy (here in particular cyproterone acetate) on the liver, we were unable to detect any indications of functional disturbances or alterations in the sense of neoplasias, as it was already the case in other investigations [9] of high-dose oral cyproterone acetate application over many years. All liver parameters and the findings of noninvasive ultrasonographic investigations were within normal ranges.

This does not eliminate the obligation to monitor carefully patients under high-dose hormone therapy, as in CPA application in hirsutism. In suspicious cases, ultrasonography is a control method which constitutes a small burden to the patient.

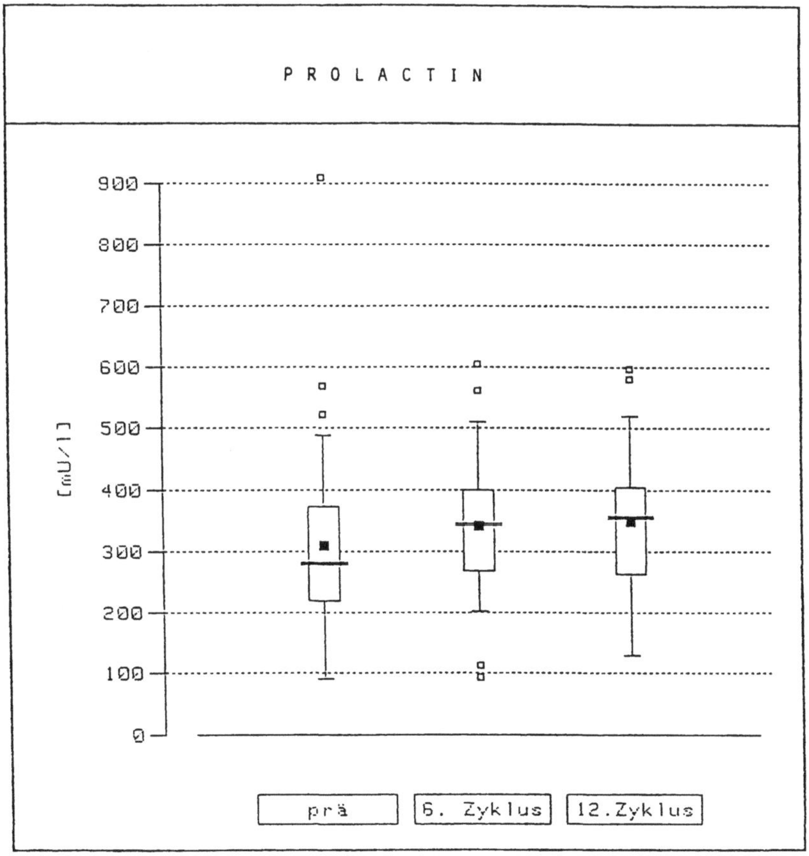

Fig. 14

The mechanism of the favorable therapeutic effect of moderately high-dose parenteral application of cyproterone acetate is not yet clear. According to Moltz et al. [13], pharmacokinetic data can not provide an explanation. These investigators found very much higher half maximal plasma levels after daily oral administration of 100 mg cyproterone acetate than after a single injection of 300 mg cyproterone acetate over the period of 10 to 12 days. Increased accumulations in the skin were found only with oral administration [15]. Since one of the metabolites of cyproterone acetate also shows antiandrogenic activity, it is conceivable that the two application forms differ with regard to metabolism. Another possibility is that the constant availability from the depot leads to greater efficacy of antiandrogenic action of the active substance at the target organ than is the case with the greater fluctuations in cyproterone acetate levels after daily oral application.

The experience communicated by urologists in antiandrogenic therapy of prostate carcinoma [10] and the reports on use of cyproterone acetate to suppress drive in sexual deviations [11] which is available from psychiatrists also show that the dose of Androcur® Depot per unit of time which is required to attain clinical effects comparable to those achieved with oral Androcur® Depot medication is smaller.

It remains an open question as to why only about 70% of the women with androgenetic androgenization symptoms show a satisfactory response to antiandrogen therapy. Pharmaco-genetic factors can postulated as a possible cause.

To summarize, equally good therapeutic results could be obtained in patients with severe androgenization symptoms using Androcur® Depot i. m. administered together with Diane® in the reverse sequential scheme and using the high-dose oral scheme we have used so far. It was our impression that tolerance was if anything better in the group of patients treated according to the new scheme for one year which can be reviewed up to now. The acceptance of parenteral cyproterone acetate application was good. In our opinion, it thus constitutes an alternative for the treatment of pronounced androgenization symptoms, which is worth consideration.

References

[1] Fixson, U.: Vorläufige Mitteilung über ein neues oral wirksames Gestagen (SH 714). Geburtsh. u. Frauenheilk. **23** (1963) 371.

[2] Flückiger, R., E. del Poso, K. von Werder: Prolactin. Monographs on Endocrinology, Vol. 23, pp. 119. Springer, Berlin—Heidelberg—New York 1982.

[3] Frölich, M., H. L. Vader, S. T. Walma et al.: The influence of longterm treatment with cyproterone acetate or a cyproterone acetate-ethinyl estradiol combination on androgen levels in blood of hirsute women. J. Steroid Biochem. **12** (1980) 499.

[4] Hammerstein, J., B. Cupceancu: Behandlung des Hirsutismus mit Cyproteronacetat. Dtsch. med. Wsch. **94** (1969) 829.

[5] Hammerstein, J., J. Meckies, I. Leo-Roßberg et al.: Use of cyproterone acetate (CPA) in the treatment of acne, hirsutism and virilism. J. Steroid Biochem. **6** (1975) 827.

[6] Kaiser, E., E.-G. Loch, G. Winckelmann et al.: Antiandrogene Behandlung bei Akne u. Hirsutismus. Med. Welt **27** (1976) 1836.

[7] Kaiser, E.: Antiandrogene Behandlung bei Akne, Haarausfall und Hirsutismus. Münch. med. Wschr. **122** (1980) 975.

[8] Kaiser, E.: Androgenisierungserscheinung der Frau. Medical Cosmotelogy (ISBN 3 7650 16683) Braun, G., Karlsruhe 1985.

[9] Kaiser, E., H. J. Gruner: Ultrasonographische Befunde der Leber und biochemische Leberparameter unter Langzeitbehandlung mit Cyproteronacetat. (In Vorbereitung.)

[10] Klosterhalfen, H., H. Becker: Antiandrogen therapy of prostatic carcinoma. Clinical experience with Androcur®/Androcur®-Depot. In: Klosterhalfen, H. (ed.): The therapy of advanced carcinoma of the prostate, pp. 63—65, Medico-scientific book series of Schering AG West Germany, Berlin 1984.

[11] Laschet, U., L. Laschet: Ten years cyproterone acetate for modification of sexual behavior in men. bga-Berichte 3/78.

[12] Moltz, L., U. Schwartz, J. Hammerstein: Die klinische Anwendung von Antiandrogenen bei der Frau. Gynäkologe **13** (1980) 1.

[13] Moltz, L., F. Haase, U. Schwartz et al.: Die Behandlung androgenisierter Frauen mit intramuskulär applizierbarem Cyproteronacetat. Geburtsh. u. Frauenheilk. **43** (1983) 281.

[14] Neumann, F.: Klinik der Antiandrogene. Dtsch. Ärzteblatt **75** (1978) 1633.

[15] Schmidt, A.: CPA-Konzentrationsbestimmungen in der Haut und im Plasma androgenisierter Frauen. Inauguraldissertation. Freie Universität Berlin 1983.

[16] Winkler, K., H. Schaefer: Verhalten der Talgsekretion während Behandlung der Acne mit Cyproteronacetat und Aethinyloestradiol. Arch. Derm. Forsch. **247** (1973) 259.

One-year experience with a new oral contraceptive using natural estradiol and cyproterone acetate

E. Hirvonen, U.-H. Stenman, E. Vartiainen

Introduction

Since risk of thrombotic and atherosclerotic complications among the users of oral contraceptives increases with age particularly in smoking women, oral contraceptives are not generally recommended to women over 40. IUDs are not accepted in all countries and sterilization is not acceptable to all women. Therefore the need of noninvasive reversible contraceptive method free from risk of cardiovascular complications is evident.

Fertility of woman begins to decline after 35 and hormonal disturbances typical to this age appear. This means that reasonable good contraceptive results can be obtained with less potent agents than contained in the usual oral contraceptives. It is desirable that oral contraceptives for women between the age of 35 and menopause have beneficial effects on dysfunctional bleeding, premenstrual tension, dysmenorrhea and skin disorders and a preventive effect against extra-uterine pregnancy, functional ovarian cysts and pelvic imflammatory disease and free from any adverse effects on blood coagulation mechanism, lipoproteins and blood pressure [1].

Natural estradiol-17-β-valerate (Progynova®) has been widely used for postmenopausal replacement therapy without any serious side-effects whereas trials to use it as a component of oral contraceptives have not succeeded because of poor cycle control. Of the 17-α-OH-progesterone derivatives only cyproterone acetate is used in oral contraceptives (Diane®). This substance is better known as a potent antiandrogen but it is also a strong progestin with a great gonadotropin inhibiting effect. The steroid content of the modern oral contraceptives has been decreased without deterioration of the cycle control. This has been managed by using the new bi- and triphasic formulations (Triquilar®).

With these facts in mind we designed two biphasic formulations using natural estradiol combined with either cyproterone acetate or norethisterone and gave them to ovulating women of 35 to 47 years of age.

Patients and methods

Fifty healthy ovulating women without other contraceptive precautions between age 35 and 47 (mean 39) underwent double-blind randomization into two groups receiving either estradiol valerate/cyproterone acetate combination (group A) or estradiol valerate/norethisterone combination (group B) (fig. 1) for six months. After these six months the study was continued in an open design. The participants were required to visit the clinic at days 12, 14, 16 and 22 of the pretreatment cycle and of the 1st, 3rd, and 6th treatment cycles. Furthermore on day 22 of the 9th and 12th treatment cycles blood samples for determination of serum FSH, LH, PRL, estradiol and estrone, progesterone and SHBG were taken. Serum was stored at 24°C until assayed with radioimmunoassay methods. Fasting blood samples were taken twice with special technique for coagulation studies during the pretreatment cycle and in the end of the 1st and 3rd treatment cycles. Lipoproteins were also measured twice during pretreatment cycle and then every 3rd month. Diary cards were issued to the participants to record withdrawal and intermenstrual bleedings, intensity of bleedings and side effects. Weight and blood pressure were recorded every 3rd month.

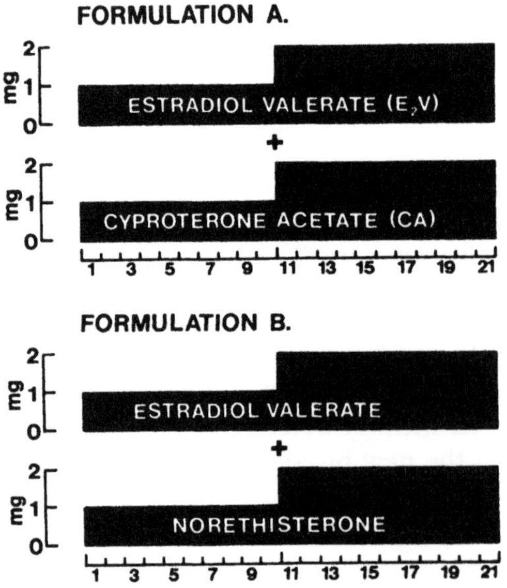

Fig. 1 Design of the formulations

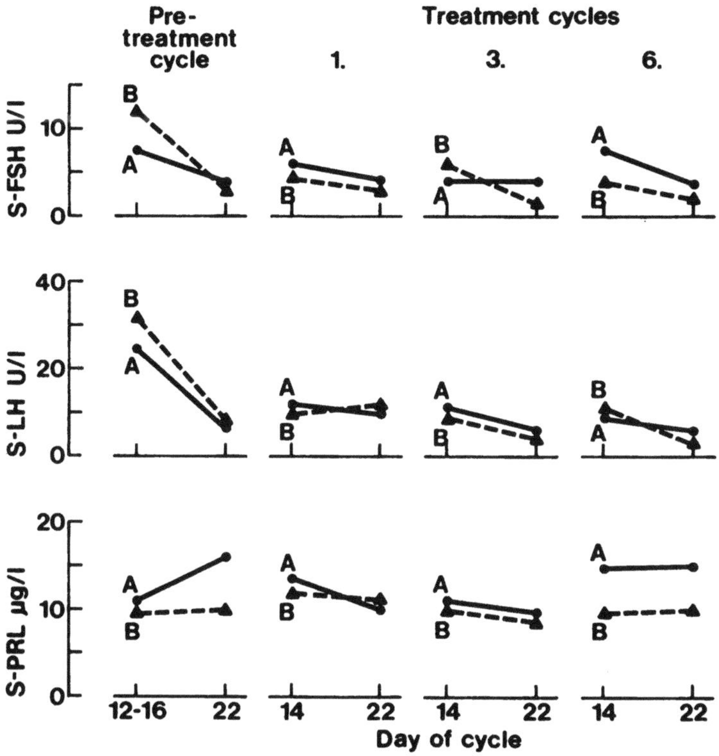

Fig. 2 S-FSH, s-LH and s-PRL concentrations before and during treatment with estradiol valerate/cyproterone acetate combination (A) and with estradiol valerate/norethisterone combination (B).

Results

Mid-cycle serum FSH and LH-peaks were suppressed but the mid-luteal values as well as prolactin were not affected (fig. 2). Compared to the pretreatment values estradiol values did not change but estrone levels increased by 2- to 4-fold (fig. 3). SHBG concentration showed a slight increase in group A and a tendency to decrease in group B. Serum progesterone values indicate that only one ovulatory cycle occurred during the first year in group A while 11 occurred in group B (tab. 1). No significant changes except an increase of plasminogen ($p<0.05$) were observed in 12 coagulation factors which were measured in 16 women in group A (tab. 2). Serum total cholesterol concentration decreased by 9 per cent ($p<0.001$) in group A and by 11 per cent in group B ($p<0.001$) and HDL-cholesterol concentration decreased by 12 per cent in group B ($p<0.001$) but did not change for six months in group A.

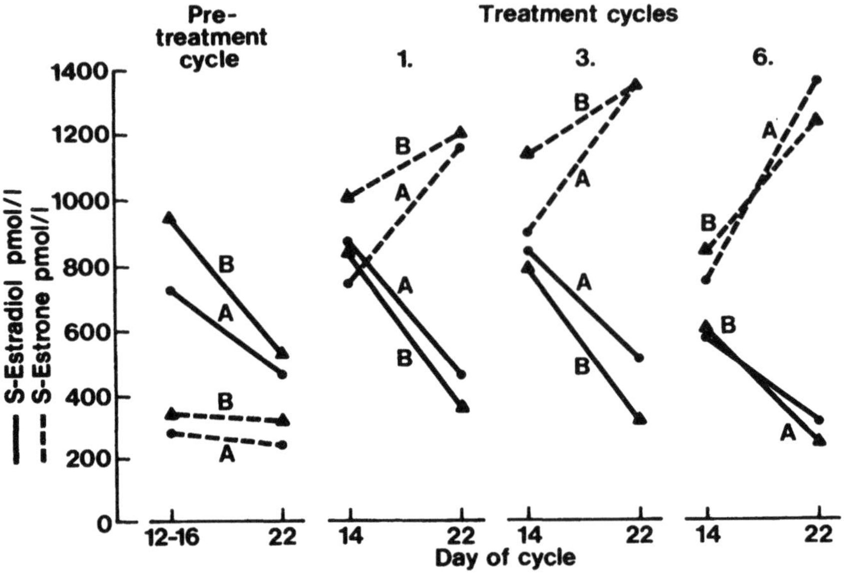

Fig. 3 S-estradiol and s-estrone concentrations during pre-treatment and 1st, 3rd and 6th treatment cycles.

Table 1 S-progesterone values (nmol/l) and number of ovulations before and during treatment

Cycle	Group A S-progesterone	Ovulations	Group B S-progesterone	Ovulations
Pre-treatment	38.2 ± 15.1	26	38.8 ± 18.5	24
1st treatment	3.1 ± 3.3	1	6.4 ± 7.6	4
3rd treatment	1.9 ± 1.6	0	3.7 ± 4.2	2
6th treatment	2.1 ± 1.1	0	7.8 ± 9.2	5
9th treatment	2.0 ± 1.1	0	2.1 ± 2.1	0
12th treatment	1.7 ± 0.7	0	2.1 ± 0.9	0

Table 2 Coagulation parameters before and during treatment with estradiol valerate/cyproterone acetate combination in 16 women in group A

Cycle	Fibri-nogen (g/l)	P and P (%)	APTT (sec)	F VIII: C (%)	AT III (mg/100 ml)	Plasmino-gen (mg/100 ml)	Protein C
Pre-treatment	2.5	95.5	40.4	55.3	104	103.4	99.9
1st treatment	2.8	100.1	40.1	55.6	102	111.0	95.9
3rd treatment	2.6	108.1	38.7	52.7	101	108.8	95.9

The heavy bleedings which were present in 8 women in group A decreased in all except in one woman with uterine fibromas. This patient had to give up the treatment after three months because of breakthrough bleeding. In contrast four women in group B withdrew from the trial because of breakthrough bleeding.

The incidence of spotting varied between 20 and 40 per cent but the total number of all bleeding days per cycle including spotting decreased in group A and remained unchanged in group B (tab. 3). One subject in group A suffered from depression but none complained of the decrease of libido. The most common side-effect was discomfort in the breasts (tab. 4) which, however, decreased during the second half of the treatment. Only three subjects in group A and five in group B discontinued the treatment because of side-effects (tab. 5). The degree of satisfaction was quite high. At the end of the first treatment year 81 per cent in group A and 67 per cent in group B were willing to go on with the treatment.

Table 3 Average number of bleeding days per cycle (mean ± S.D.)

	Pre-treatment	3rd	6th	9th	12th
A	5.0 ± 1.0	5.8 ± 4.0	5.2 ± 3.7	3.7 ± 2.3	4.0 ± 3.1
B	4.9 ± 1.2	5.9 ± 3.3	4.9 ± 1.6	5.1 ± 2.3	5.2 ± 2.5

Table 4 Side-effects

	Pre-treatment		3rd treatment		6th treatment		12th treatment	
	A	B	A	B	A	B	A	B
Headache	2	0	8	2	6	3	4	2
Oedema	7	9	8	6	4	4	3	1
Breast tension	3	1	17	11	8	8	6	3
Depression	1	0	7	1	2	1	0	1

Table 5 Reasons for discontinuation of the trial

	Number of subjects	Completed cycles	Reason for discontinuation
Group A	1	3	BTB (fibromas)
	1	4	Desire of pregnancy
	1	6	Varicose complaints
	1	9	Spotting, depression
Group B	4	3, 6, 6, 9	Spotting + BTB
	1	2	Oedema, weight gain
	1	8	Desire of pregnancy
	2	6, 7	Medical reason

Discussion

The combination estradiol valerate/cyproterone acetate achieved better clinical results. The cycle control was tolerable and bleedings became scant. This is probably explained by the longer half-life of cyproterone acetate compared to that of norethisterone [3] and more effective down-regulation of estrogen receptors. Disappearance of dysmenorrhea is obviously due to similar mechanism as during treatment with usual oral contraceptives. Serum estrone values increase when estradiol is given orally [4] and in this study they reflect the dose of estradiol given per day better than the estradiol values of which a part is endogenous explaining the similar serum estradiol values during pretreatment and treatment cycles.

The almost total inhibition of ovulation in group A, which received the estradiol valerate/cyproterone acetate combination, indicates that this combination is safe in this age group. Furthermore, absence of effect on coagulation parameters and on HDL-cholesterol level may indicate that it has neither trombogenic nor atherogenic risks. It can also be used in the treatment of dysmenorrhea and dysfunctional bleedings. According to our experience it is useful in the treatment of hyperandrogenic symptoms such as acne and seborrhea in older women and in those who complain of side-effects from ethinyl estradiol. Also the combination of cyproterone acetate in reversal system [2] has shown to be possible.

References

[1] Guillebaud, J.: Contraception for the older woman. J. Ostet. Gynaecol. **5** (1985) 70—77.
[2] Hammerstein, J.: Possibilities and limits of endocrine therapy. In: Hammerstein, J., U. Lachnit-Fixon (eds.): Androgenization in women, pp. 221—238. Excerpta Medica, Amsterdam—Oxford—Princeton 1980.
[3] Humpel, M., H. Wendt, G. Dogs et al.: Intraindividual comparison of pharmacokinetic parameters of D-norgestrel, lynestrenol and cyproterone acetate in 6 women. Contraception **16** (1977) 199—202.
[4] Yen, SSC., P. Martin, A. Burnier et al.: Circulating estradiol, estrone and gonadotropin levels following the administration of orally active 17-β-estradiol in postmenopausal women. J. Clin. Endocrinol. Metab. **40** (1975) 518—522.

Discussion

Spona: This afternoon session highlighted some clinical aspects of side effects and the application of cyproterone acetate.

I take the chairman's priviledge to open the discussion and ask Dr. Bruni: Do you have any data comparing antithrombin III in women taking either Diane® or Diane-35®?

Bruni: No, I have no data on the changes in the haemostatic system under Diane® available. We compared Diane-35® versus two triphasic preparations containing either levonorgestrel or gestoden. We saw no differences in the coagulation parameters between the two triphasic preparations. But it would be extremely interesting to compare Diane® and Diane-35®, two preparations with the same gestagen and different ethinyl estradiol content.

Silverstolpe: Effects on the coagulation factors from exogenous sex steroids are likely to appear quickly often within weeks. On Diane-35® you found after 6 cycles of treatment a 30% increase of antithrombin III (AT III) activity. This is surprising since one would have expected an effect much earlier if there was an effect. Ethinyl estradiol even in low doses such as 10 μg is known to decrease AT III activity. Is your observation an effect of cyproterone acetate?

Bruni: Yes, I believe that the increase of AT III is a direct effect of cyproterone acetate, because we did not see similar changes under the intake of other gestagens. The other gestagens showed the expected decrease of AT III. We contribute the effect of cyproterone acetate to its antiandrogenic activity. We controlled our results after a longer time of treatment and found our results confirmed after twelve and fifteen months.

Schindler: For the evaluation of the side effects of a combination of an antiandrogen and an estrogen or any other combination pill it seems to be important to look simultaneously on the coagulation factors on the one side — and on the fibrinolytic activity on the other side. Would you like to comment on that?

Bruni: No, I do not believe that the hypothesis of the balance between the coagulation factors and the fibrinolytic activity is a satisfaying solution to the problem. Because we do not know whether the coagulation factors are really the only important ones for the thromboembolic risk. For this reason we have used pregnant women as a physiological model to evaluate the effects of gestagens. In our study of 20 healthy women with uncomplicated pregnancies we found a significant reduction of the fibrinolytic activities. Therefore the evaluation of the stabilization of the haemostatic system is very difficult, because there are many so far unknown factors like anticortison, antiestrogens and other factors acting directly at the vessel wall. But as I mentioned a combination preparation raising the coagulation factors and raising AT III as an indicator for the activated fibrinolytic activity means an ideal pill combination in my opinion.

Gaspard: I have seen with interest that you saw a decrease of fibrinolytic activity when you are performing a venous occlusion during the treatment with Diane-35®. Did you see the same type of decrease in fibrinolytic activity in the control group, patients not taking this preparation? Do you have an explanation for this? We personally have seen during venous occlusion under the intake of triphasic contraceptives an increase in the alpha-20-plasmin. Could there be a relationship between your observation and ours?

Bruni: Sorry, you did not understand my slides correctly. We did not see a decrease of fibrinolytic activity, we saw however an increase, a mechanism we cannot interpret. A reduction of fibrinolytic activity could only be seen in a combination of 50 mg EE and 100 mg cyproterone acetate and in men, taking 10 mg cyproterone acetate daily.

Cohen: I want to ask Dr. Ernst, whether he saw an effect of smoking on rheology.

Ernst: There are plenty of data showing the effects of smoking. But in our own studies we could not find any effect of age on rheology.

It would be of interest in this context to see whether the addition of smoking and contraceptive pill does have some potentiating effect, but we have not studied this.

Spona: Dr. Ashton presented a very interesting paper on the treatment of acne patients. Are there any questions on this subject?

Nuernberger: Did you add an additional local treatment?

Ashton: Most of our patients enrolled in this study were all patients who had previous acne treatment by their family doctors, most of them had topical treatment as well as systemic antibiotic treatment. They have failed and hence they have been referred to further specialist advice to our skin department.

Except for contraceptive pills they had no treatment of any kind for 6 weeks prior to the entrance into the study.

Spona: You made a very interesting statement, that you did not find any correlation between the clinical improvement, sebum excretion rate (SER) and testosterone serum levels. Does that mean you had high testosterone serum levels in patients who responded as well as in patients who did not respond to the treatment? And the same is true for sebum excretion rate?

Ashton: Yes, basicly we saw no correlation between the severity of acne and the elevation of testosterone and SER.

Falsetti: I want to point out, that you measured only the total testosterone and not the free testosterone. May be this is the explanation why you did not find a correlation.

Ashton: We measured both the total and the free testosterone and both total and free dihydrotestosterone and there was no correlation in all the parameters studied.

Lachnit: I suggest, that the fact that most of your patients had almost normal free and total testosterone values is due to the fact that they where continuing oral contraceptives still before starting treatment. We know that any normal oral contraceptive pill has the ability to decrease total and free testosterone. That might be the explanation for your missing correlation.

And I also want to point out again to what Prof. Neumann already mentioned this morning, that a preparation like Diane-35® has a dual effect: First by inhibition of the ovulation and second by the peripheral antiandrogenic effect at the receptor site at the target organ.

Ashton: I would agree. I am a dermatologist and therefore interested in the skin. And the skin is an end organ for androgens. This is an end organ problem. It does seem from the results of our study that hormonal levels in the blood are not so important as perhaps the response of the skin, i.e. the end organ response.

Rubens: Could you tell something about the relapse rate?

Ashton: I think there is no good study showing how long you should continue the Diane® treatment and what the relapse rate will be. I think especially that the decrease of ethinyl estradiol in Diane-35® will allow continuing for a longer treatment, perhaps 18 to 24 months.

Spona: I want to make a short comment. I fully agree with the end organ sensitivity. What is then your explanation for the effect on the bacterial counts?

Ashton: The decrease of the bacterial counts was more pronounced than the improvement of the sebum excretion rate. The bacteria are certainly a secondary phenomen. When the acne becomes better, the altering environment for the bacteria seems to drop down the bacterial counts.

Bruni: I may be allowed to add a short comment. Personally I do not believe, that acne is only an endocrinological problem. Acne is more a problem of the skin—a dermatosis. Therefore you get an ideal effect by combining endocrinological and local, i.e. dermatological therapy.

Ashton: When talking about the pustles of acne I suppose there are two main things: first there is the sebum excretion rate and second there is the blockage of the pores. There is no doubt that sebum excretion rate is androgen dependent, even if not totally.

It is interesting, that in the first group of our patients, who did not take cyproterone acetate, the sebum excretion rate did not actually decrease very much although the acne itself became better. Then you have this problem with the blockage of the pores. There again one does not know the part, which the androgens play, whether they alter the cohesiveness of the cells or what else.

Spona: A very short and final comment on the subject. It is certainly very much endocrine dependent, because you can show by topical active androgenic treatment that you achieve a very good result. So there is at least a high control on the end organ sensitivity of the skin, which is an endocrine organ.

Cohen: Then we want to discuss the paper of Dr. Rubens. I may ask the first question. You had so many patients with tiredness with cyproterone acetate. Do you have any idea why?

Rubens: No, I have none. But if you start asking them whether they have noted tiredness and whether they have the same muscular ability than they had before the treatment, you will end up with many positive answers. I think it is quite explainable. If athlets get androgens to have higher muscular performance and you give people antiandrogens they will have less muscular performance. That seems quite explainable to me.

Kaiser: Why did you give the spironolactone in cyclic manner? I saw this also on the slide of Prof. Schindler's lecture this morning. In our outpatient clinic we see many patients with hypertention. We also treat them with spironolactone 100 mg and more contineously and we never saw menstrual cycle disturbances.

Rubens: I have two reasons for the cyclic manner of application of spironolactone:

1. About 6 years ago Bots and Shane published their trials in rhesus monkeys proving a very slight gestagenic effect of spironolactone.
2. In the original papers from Roussell and Shapiro they have reported cyclic disturbances.

Spona: The next paper that is open for the discussion is that of Dr. Kaiser, who showed some interesting data on intramuscular application of cyproterone acetate. I noted you found a better therapy by the intramusculary treatment compared with the oral treatment. I am very interested in that, because we have the same results. We looked at the cyproterone acetate levels in serum and found no different pharmacokinetic data. Do you have any explanation for your data, where you got the better therapy results in the intramusculary treated patients?

Kaiser: No, at the moment we have no acceptable explanation for this.

Cohen: We are going to the last speaker, to the very interesting investigation of Dr. Hirvonen. I have three questions. The first question: Where is the origin of your data on the fertility of premenopausal women of 40 and 45 years. You mentioned a fertility of about 20%, which in my experience is too high.

Hirvonen: I referred to a paper of Killeborgs published 1981 in the Journal of Gynecology and Obstetrics.

Cohen: My second question is: You proposed this kind of contraception with estradiol valerate and cyproterone acetate just because the fertility of that age is reduced. Does this mean, that if we gave the same kind of oral contraceptive pill to a younger women perhaps 30 years, we could have pregnancies?

Hirvonen: No, I do not think so. We have not tried this combination in younger women, because we just were not sure about the ovulation inhibiting effect of this combination. Therefore we started the trial with older women. But now we are convinced that it could be a safe preparation also in younger women.

Cohen: My last question is: Why did you try with the progressive dose of estradiol valerate and why did you not take a constant combination all over the cycle?

Hirvonen: We thought that this biphasic manner of application could improve cycle control.

Schindler: But you have not been very successful regarding this prevention of intermenstrual bleedings, when I look at your data. You argue now that you have used a biphasic preparation, you should better say a step-up method, because you stepped up in both estrogens and gestagens. My question would be: have you ever tried a combination of 2 mg EV and 2 mg cyproterone acetate over 21 days?

Hirvonen: No, we have not. But we have given it in a reverse manner, starting with the tablet with a higher amount of estradiol valerate, but the spotting problems in these patients were the same. I think, it should also be noted that the selection of patients for our study was relative negative. Many of them had hypermenorrhoe and bleeding problems under the IUD, some of them had intermenstrual bleedings. All the intermenstrual bleedings were not strong only spotting and after the first year the spotting rate decreased to 10%.

What I found out which is more interesting, that the spotting rates under the combination of estradiol valerate and norethisterone were much higher.

Schindler: This does not astonish me at all. Because when you compare equal amounts of norethisterone and cyproterone acetate I know from another study of mine, that the hydroxyprogesterone derivates, such as cyproterone acetate will be superior to norethisterone regarding the effect on the endometrium. And therefore we can state again, coming back to our morning discussion that we should not only use the progesterone derivates for the postmenopausal, but we should also go forward and prefer the hydroxyprogesterone preparations even in the premenopausal women.

Cohen: Yes, I would agree. May be that we shall step even more forward up to puberty. I want to close this afternoon session and thank all the speakers and all the participants in the audience.

V Metabolic and clinical aspects

Clinical and metabolic effects of a new estrogen-antiandrogen low dose combination

L. De Cecco, G. L. Capitanio, S. Bertolini, S. Croce, A. Centonze

Introduction

It has long been recognized that the use of cyproterone acetate (CPA) as a monophasic or inversally sequential combination with ethinyl estradiol (EE) for contraception and treatment in women with slight or moderate clinical signs of hyperandrogenism because of multifollicular ovary proves to be clinically useful.

However, in the above-mentioned combination a dosage of 50 mcg of ethinyl estradiol has always been employed.

Thereafter, the clinical and metabolic effects of a new monophasic combination containing cyproterone acetate with low-dose (35 mcg) ethinyl estradiol were investigated.

Material and methods

Twenty-four healthy young women (age: 25.9 ± 6.6 years) were selected from a group of patients requiring basic contraceptive treatment for some clinical features (acne, seborrhea, moderate hypertrichosis or hirsutism) showing a situation of a slight to moderate hyperandrogenism.

The patients were treated over six cycles with monophasic combination of 0.035 mg of ethinyl estradiol (EE) and 2 mg of cyproterone acetate (CPA) for 21 consecutive days.

The first treatment cycle was started on the first day of bleeding: between each cycle and the next one a seven-day discontinuation period was performed.

The subjects were studied in basal conditions (luteal phase)—any previous oral contraceptive treatment having been discontinued 3 months before at least—and after 2, 4 and 6 cycles.

Plasma concentrations of total cholesterol (Tc), LDL-cholesterol (LDLc), HDL-cholesterol (HDLc) and its fractions HDL_2 and HDL_3 (HDL_2c, HDL_3c), triglycerides (TG), apoproteins A_I, A_{II}, B, C_{II}, C_{III}, E (Apo A_I, Apo_{II}, Apo B,

Apo C_{II}, Apo C_{III}, Apo E), body weight (kg) and blood pressure (SBP, DBP) were checked at each visit.

At follow-up examination the patients were questioned about the onset and extent of side-effects and the control of cycles. Moreover, they were asked about a personal assessment of drug influence on seborrhea and acne.

Blood samples were taken after an overnight fast (12—14 h) between the 21st and the 25th day of the menstrual cycle (basal conditions) and on the day after the 19th and the 21st day of treatment cycles.

Lipoprotein determinations

For lipoprotein assay the blood was taken using multisample needles (Terumo MN-2038M) and evacuated tubes (Terumo venojets VT 050Na) containing 7.5 mg of EDTA-Na (final. conc. 1.5 mg/ml of blood); cells were removed (within 20 minutes) by low-speed centrifugation (1500 × g for 30 minutes at 4° C) and the plasma samples were kept at 4° C until analysis always performed, for the lipids, within 4 hours from blood taking.

Tc, HDLc, HDL_3c and TG were assayed by enzymatic methods using commercial kits (Monotest, Cholesterol High Performance, CHOD-PAP method, Boehringer Mannheim GmbH cat. n. 237574 and Test Combination Triglycerides GPO-PAP High Performance, Boehringer Mannheim GmbH cat. n. 701912).

HDLc was determined in the supernatant after precipitation from the whole plasma of Apo B containing lipoproteins (VLDL, LDL) by heparin (sodium salt, Sigma grade 1, 178 USP/mg. cat. n. H-3125) and $MnCl_2$ (final concentrations 184 U/ml and 92 mmol/L respectively).

HDL_2 and HDL_3 subfractions were separated by the method of Gidez et al. [1]: HDL_3c was quantified in the supernatant after precipitation from the heparin-Mn^{2+} supernatant of the HDL_2 subfraction by Dextran Sulphate 15000 m.w.; HDL_2c was obtained by subtracting HDL_3 from total HDLc.

HDL_3c determination was performed immediately after HDL_2 precipitation to assure the best correlation with the values obtained by sequential ultracentrifugation [2].

No interference on enzymatic analysis of HDLc because of residual Mn^{2+} ions was found: the accuracy of the assay was checked using the chemical extraction method of Abell et al. [3] ($r = 0.993$) and treating heparin-Mn^{2+} supernatant with $NaHCO_3$ (final concentration 91 mmol/L) to precipitate Mn^{2+} as suggested by Bachorik et al. [4] (absorbance at 830 nm) as index of turbidity was 0.013 ± 0.002 for 100 mcL heparin-Mn^{2+} supernatant untreated + 900 mcL enzymic reagent buffer and 0.014 ± 0.002 for 100 mcL heparin-Mn^{2+} supernatant treated with $NaHCO_3$ + 900 mcL enzymic reagent buffer ($n = 10$).

LDLc was calculated using Friedwald's formula [5]:

$$LDLc = Tc - HDLc - TG/5$$

Plasma samples for Apoprotein assays were kept at $-30°C$; the determinations were made by Radial Immunodiffusion Method (Daichi Plates, Daichi Pure Chemicals Co., Ltd, Tokyo; Cu% 2.5—3.5).

Clinical results

No pregnancy occured during the treatment of the 24 subjects. All the patients took the preparation regularely with no omission.

Spotting was reported in 37.5% (n=9) at the end of 2nd cycle, in 25% (n=6) at the end of 4th cycle, in 4% (n=1) at the end of the 6th cycle. During the 6th treatment cycle no episode was reported. No breakthrough bleeding was reported.

The most frequent side-effects were:

— headache (4.1%, n=6),
— mastodynia (5%, n=7),
— nausea/vomiting (2%, n=3),
— feeling of heaviness at legs (5%, n=7),
— increase in body weight (8.3%, n=10).

The percentage incidence of side-effects is given on the total number of cycles; this incidence regards mainly the first treatment cycles and decreased progressively except for body weight. No side-effect caused treatment discontinuation. Patients evaluation of therapeutic effect of the drug is summarized in table 1. Systolic and diastolic arterial pressure value remained practically unchanged.

Table 1 Patients evaluation of therapeutic effects

		2nd cycle	4th cycle	6th cycle
		number of patients		
FATTY SKIN (n = 24)	unchanged	5	3	2
	slightly improved	16	13	8
	considerably improved	3	8	14
ACNE (n = 24)	unchanged	12	8	4
	slightly improved	8	12	14
	considerably improved	4	4	6
FATTY HAIR (n = 24)	unchanged	4	2	1
	slightly improved	16	13	6
	considerably improved	4	9	17
HAIR LOSS (n = 16)	unchanged	13	10	6
	slightly improved	3	6	9
	considerably improved	–	–	1

Table 2 Values as mean ± standard deviation in mg/dl (^{ns} = non significant)

	Baseline	2nd cycle	4th cycle	6th cycle
TC	154.1 ±17.6	167.1 ±21.4*	171.3 ±32.6^{ns}	171.4 ±28.3*
LDL_c	88.1 ±15.4	85.3 ±22.3^{ns}	89.3 ±32.2^{ns}	87.5 ±26.3^{ns}
TG	66.2 ±15.6	106.3 ±29.3***	106.7 ±37.1***	114.3 ±37.8***
HDL_c	52.7 ± 7.1	60.6 ± 6.2***	60.7 ± 9.3***	61.0 ± 8.3***
HDL_{2c}	17.1 ± 3.9	21.8 ± 4.5***	21.7 ± 4.9***	21.8 ± 4.7***
HDL_{3c}	35.7 ± 4.7	38.7 ± 2.1*	39.0 ± 4.6*	39.2 ± 3.9**
LDL_c/HDL_c	1.70± 0.39	1.44± 0.51*	1.52± 0.62^{ns}	1.47± 0.49^{ns}
Kg	53.6 ± 7.0	54.4 ± 7.1^{ns}	54.7 ± 7.8*	55.1 ± 7.5*
Apo A I	139.0 ±16.4			176.0 ±13.0***
Apo A II	27.9 ± 4.6			42.0 ± 4.2***
Apo C II	2.62± 0.6			3.37± 0.85***
Apo C III	7.27± 1.64			10.40± 2.57***
Apo B	66.2 ±13.2			89.8 ±15.6***
Apo E	3.62± 0.81			3.46± 0.92^{ns}

* $p<0.05$ ** $p<0.01$ *** $p<0.001$

Changes in lipoprotein metabolism

The results, given as mean values upon completion of 2nd, 4th and 6th treatment cycle, are summarized in table 2. The significance of results vs baseline values was calculated by Student's test for paired data.

Discussion

a) Clinical results

In the 24 patients of our study complete contraceptive effectiveness, good tolerance with improvement in the course of treatment and good cycle control were observed following drug intake.

The non-contraceptive therapeutical effect with correction of the slight absolute or relative hyperandrogenism of the patients, probably affected with initial phases of multi-follicular ovary syndrome, proved to be definitely satisfactory.

Most patients (tab. 1) passed a positive judgement on almost all the symptoms of hyperandrogenism complained of at admission. Body weight increase was moderate and kept within limits regarded as acceptable for a low-dose estrogen-antiandrogen treatment.

b) Lipo-apolipo-protein changes

Before taking into account the metabolic effects of the preparation a preliminary consideration has to be made as to the basic metabolic features of the patients of our study. There are some features of the basal lipoprotein pattern which do reflect clearly enough the situation of slight hyperandrogenism already shown at the previous clinical screening. The HDL (HDLc, HDL_2, HDL_3, Apo A_I) system, highly responsive to an even slightly hyperandrogenic situation, appears to be influenced with values decisively inferior to those usually found in healthy young women, even though still within normal limits.

The slightly androgenic profile of the patients was not however such as to influence also the basal values of VLDL-LDL system and its related apoproteins (mainly Apo B), less easily responsive to both endogenous androgenic influences and the treatment with androgens and/or androgenic progestagens.

The estrogenic/antiandrogenic effect of the combination under trial clearly stands out at the level of all lipoprotein and apolipo-protein fractions.

In particular, there is a clear-cut corrective effect of the treatment on the HDL-Apo A_I system with a statistically significant increase ($p<0.001$) starting from 2nd cycle, continuing over the whole treatment duration and involving both the whole HDLc fraction and HDL_2c subfraction.

The increase in all the Apoproteins (A_I, A_{II}, C_{II}, C_{III}) related to the HDL system bears out their activation degree both as liver synthesis of nascent apoproteins [6] and HDL as well as an increased conversion rate of HDL_3 into HDL_2 (increase in adipose lipoproteinlipase activity). Also the reduced catabolism (inhibition of hepatic lipase) [6, 7, 8] probably takes part in bringing about an increase in HDL fraction.

The increase in triglycerides (VLDL) and Apo B is likewise the attribute to the on the whole proestrogenic effect of the combination under trial. In fact, under estrogenic influence there is an increase in liver synthesis of both triglycerides and apoproteins B [6] related to VLDL-LDL system. Progestatives have a tedency to decrease the synthesis of triglycerides and Apo B [9, 10] (gestagenic or antiestrogenic effect [10]) and to speed up their catabolic conversion rate from VLDL to IDL and then to LDL (androgenic effect [7—13]), because of an increase in liver lipase [14, 15].

On the contrary, estrogens bring about a decrease in LDL cholesterol [8, 11] both by inhibiting hepatic lipase (inhibition of synthesis) and by increasing liver synthesis of receptors for LDL particles (increase in catabolism) [12]. Thereupon, a decrease in LDL cholesterol fraction might be anticipated following the treatment with ethinyl estradiol (35 mcg)/cyproterone acetate (2 mg).

The non-occurrence of such a decrease is probably to put down to such a considerable increase in triglycerides as to mask the real activation of clearance of the LDL particles by both liver and tissues. In the same way, the increase in Apoprotein B has to be attributed to the same phenomenon: as a matter of fact, Apo B could be related to VLDL.

The mean triglyceride blood levels are safely kept within normal limits and within the overall favourable range of lipo-apo-lipoprotein pattern induced by the treatment. This data, in our view, should not be regarded as atherogenic.

Conclusion

The treatment with the combination cyproterone acetate (2 mg) + ethinyl estradiol (35 mcg) showed a reliable and well tolerated contraceptive activity in our patients along with a satisfactory non-contraceptive therapeutic effect on the clinical features of slight hyperandrogenism of the patients.

Moreover, the combination under trial made it possible to correct the metabolic effects of hyperandrogenism by producing a lipo-apolipo-protein pattern showing a clear-cut antiatherogenic profile.

Since such results are obtained with a particularly low dosage of estrogen as compared with previous formulations, it is possible to combine the advantageous lipid blood level with a decrease in both thromboembolic risk and incidence of side effects.

References

[1] Gidez, L. I., G. J. Miller, M. Burstein et al.: Separation and quantitation of subclasses of human plasma high density lipoproteins by a simple precipitation procedure. J. Lipiol. Research **23** (1982) 1206—1223.

[2] Khan, S. R., R. S. Elkeles, R. Niththyananthan et al.: Analysis of high density lipoprotein subclasses by a precipitation procedure: comparison with preparative ultracentrifuge. Clin. Chim. Acta **120** (1982) 49—55.

[3] Abell, L. L., B. B. Levy, B. B. Brodie et al.: A simplified method for the estimation of total cholesterol in serum and demonstration of its specificity. J. Biol. Chem. **195** (1962) 357—366.

[4] Bachorik, P. S., R. E. Walker, D. G. Virgil: High-density-lipoprotein cholesterol in heparin-$MnCl_2$ supernates determined with the Dow Enzymatic method after precipitation of Mn^{2+} with HCO_{3-}. Clin. Chem. **30** (1984) 839—842.

[5] Friedewald, W. T., R. I. Levy, D. S. Fredrickson: Estimation of the concentration of Low-density lipoprotein cholesterol in plasma without use of the preparative ultracentrifuge. Clin. Chem. **18** (1972) 499—502.

[6] Scheefer, E. J., D. M. Foster, L. A. Zech et al.: The effects of estrogen administration on plasma lipoprotein metabolism in premenopausal females. J. Clin. Endocrinol. Metab. **57** (1983) 262—267.

[7] Tikkanen, M. J., E. A. Nikkila, T. Kuusi et al.: Effects of estradiol and levonorgestrel on lipoprotein lipids and postheparin plasma lipase activities in normolipoprotaeinemic women. Acta Endocr. **99** (1982) 630—635.

[8] Hazzard, W. R., S. M. Hafner, R. S. Kushwaha et al.: Preliminary report: chinetic studies on the modulation of high density lipoprotein, apolipoprotein and subfraction metabolism by sex steroids in a postmenopausal woman. Metabolism **33** (1984) 779—784.

[9] Cheng, D. C. H., B. M. Wolf: Norethindrone acetate inhibition of trigliceride synthesis and release by rat epatocytes. Atherosclerosis **46** (1983) 41—48.
[10] Khokha, R., M. Wolf: Hypotriglyceridemic effects of levonorgestrel in rats. Atherosclerosis **52** (1984) 329—338.
[11] Fahraeus, L., U. Larsson-Cohn, L. Wallentin: Lipoproteins during oral and cutaneous administration of oestradiol-17 B to menopausal women. Acta Endocr. **101** (1982) 597—602.
[12] Hakes, L., T. J. C. van Berkel: In vivo characteristics of a specific recognition site for LDL on non-parenchimal rat liver cells which differs from the 17-alpha-ethinyl estradiol-induced LDL receptor on parenchymal liver cells. Biochim. Biophys. Acta **794** (1984) 340—347.
[13] Farish, E., C. D. Fletcher, D. M. Hart et al.: A long term study of the effects of norethisterone on lipoprotein metabolism in menopausal women. Clin. Chim. Acta **182** (1983) 193—198.
[14] Glueck, C. J., S. Ford, P. Steiner et al.: Triglyceride removal efficiency and lipoprotein lipases: effects of oxandrolone. Metabolism **22** (1973) 807—814.
[15] Havel, R. J.: The formation of LDL: mechanism and regulation. J. Lipid Research **25** (1984) 1570—1576.

Effects of cyproterone acetate on serum lipoproteins when administered alone and in combination with ethinyl estradiol

G. Silfverstolpe, U.-B. Lindberg, L. Enk, G. Samsioe, N. Crona

Introduction

In most oral contraceptives, ethinyl estradiol (EE) is combined with a 19-nortestosterone derivative. Both retrospective [13] and prospective studies [9] show that the progestogen component in oral contraceptives is linked to cardiovascular morbidity, possibly via the effect of this component on the lipoprotein pattern in serum. Some exogenous androgens and progestogens, which are 19-nortestosterone derivatives, decrease HDL and tend to increase LDL [4, 15]. This can adversely affect risk of coronary heart disease (CHD) [18]. Moderate oral doses of progestogens derived from 17-hydroxyprogesterone are, on the other hand, rather inert in their effects on serum lipoproteins [7, 18]. Cyproterone acetate is a 17-hydroxyprogesterone derivative which, furthermore, has certain antiandrogenic effects. Thus, it is of interest to delineate the effects on serum lipids and lipoproteins induced by cyproterone acetate, administrated alone and in combination with ethinyl estradiol.

Subjects and methods

Clinical series

21 oophorectomized women were recruited for the study. These had a mean age of 42.2 (range 33—52) years and had been operated on according to Wertheim Meigs as part of the treatment for cervical carcinoma in clinical stage IB or IIA. At least 26 months had elapsed since the operation and all women were healthy at the time of the study. No continuous medications were used among the women, eleven of whom were smokers.

Steroids studied

1. Cyproterone acetate (CPA) (1.2-methyl-ene-6-chloro-4.6-pregnandien-

17-ol.3.20-dion-17-acetate) is a 17α-hydroxyprogesterone derivative with antiandrogenic and progestational activity which is clinically exploited in the treatment of hyperandrogenic conditions such as hirsutism.

2. Ethinyl estradiol (EE), a 17-C alkylated estrogen, is the active estrogen component in all combined oral contraceptives currently available.

Study design

The study was carried out with a cross-over design (fig. 1). After a period of four weeks without any hormonal treatment, all women were given 2 mg CPA/day orally for four weeks. After this period the women were allocated to one of two groups. Nine women received 35 µg of ethinyl estradiol and twelve women received 50 µg of ethinyl estradiol added to their cyproterone acetate dose for twelve weeks. After the cross-over of the combined medication (another twelve week period) each group continued with its latest dose of ethinyl estradiol for another four week period. After the wash-out period (fig. 1) and after each treatment period, the women underwent blood sampling and physical examinations including body weight and blood pressure measurements. The blood samples were drawn from an antecubital vein in the morning after an overnight fast. To obtain serum the blood samples were centrifuged at 2.500 rpm for 10 minutes. A portion of the serum was then stored at $-20°C$. The other portion was separated by preparative ultracentrifugation into lipoprotein fractions, which were again stored at $-20°C$.

Laboratory analysis

Serum lipids: Determinations of triglycerides (TG), free and total cholesterol (FC and TC) and phospholipids (PL) were performed using commercially available kits (Boehringer-Mannheim Test No TC 237574, TC 313028, TC 126012, TC 124974.

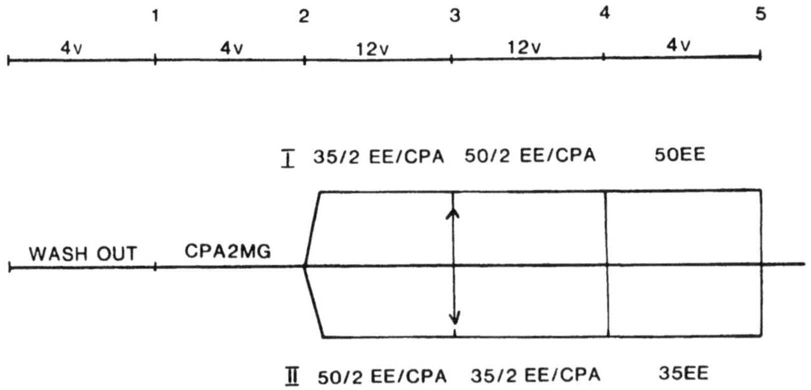

Fig. 1 Study design—see text.

Lipoprotein lipids: Preparative ultracentrifugation of serum was performed at 4°C and 105.000 × g for 22 hours in one step with a modification of the method described by Walton and coworkers using 4 ml of serum [16]. Three lipoprotein fractions were isolated: very-low-density lipoproteins (VLDL, d = 0.96—1.006 g/ml), low-density lipoproteins (LDL, d = 1.006—1.063 g/ml) and high-density lipoproteins (HDL, d = 1.063—1.21 g/ml). Within each lipoprotein fraction TG, FC, TC and PL were analysed using the methods described above.

Statistical evaluation

Evaluation was done by 2-way analysis of variance followed by the Student-Newman-Keul's multiple range test.

Results

Clinical remarks

Three women did not complete the study. No changes in blood pressure or body-weight were recorded during the study.

Serum lipids: 2 mg cyproterone acetate induced a decrease of FC ($p < 0.01$), TC ($p < 0.05$) and PL ($p < 0.05$). 2 mg cyproterone acetate in combination with 35 µg ethinyl estradiol increased TG and PL ($p < 0.01$) and concomitantly a decreased FC and TC ($p < 0.01$). The same changes were induced by 2 mg cyproterone acetate + 50 µg ethinyl estradiol.

VLDL-lipids: 2 mg cyproterone acetate alone did not induce any statistically significant changes in the VLDL fraction. 2 mg cyproterone acetate + 35 µg ethinyl estradiol increased TG, FC and PL ($p < 0.01$). The same changes were seen when 2 mg cyproterone acetate + 50 µg ethinyl estradiol were used (fig. 2).

LDL-lipids: 2 mg cyproterone acetate alone did not induce any statistically significant changes within the LDL fraction. 2 mg cyproterone acetate + 35 µg ethinyl estradiol increased TG ($p < 0.05$) and decreased FC ($p < 0.01$) and TC ($p < 0.05$). 2 mg cyproterone acetate + 50 µg ethinyl estradiol increased TG ($p < 0.05$), decreased FC and TC ($p < 0.01$) as well as PL ($p < 0.05$).

2 mg cyproterone acetate + 50 µg ethinyl estradiol induced significantly lower levels of LDL-TC and LDL-PL ($p < 0.05$) than did the administration of 2 mg cyproterone acetate + 35 µg ethinyl estradiol.

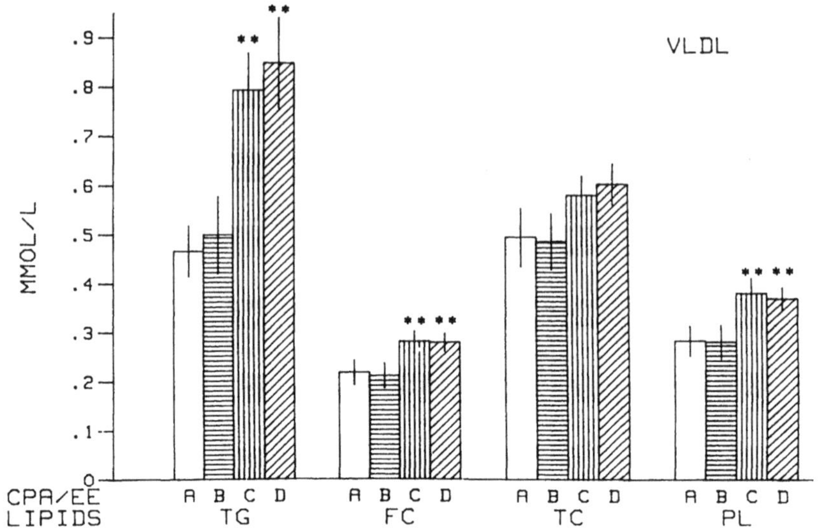

Fig. 2 Levels of lipid components in VLDL (very-low-density lipoproteins). Triglycerides (TG), free cholesterol (FC), total cholesterol (TC) and phospholipids (PL) in oophorectomized women (n = 21).
Column A—lipid level after wash-out period,
Column B—lipid level after oral administration of 2 mg CPA,
Column C—lipid level after oral administration of 2 mg CPA in combination with 35 µg EE and
Column D—lipid level after oral administration of 2 mg CPA in combination with 50 µg EE.
Asterisks indicate statistically significant changes as compared to pre-treatment values. * = $p < 0.05$; ** = $p < 0.01$.

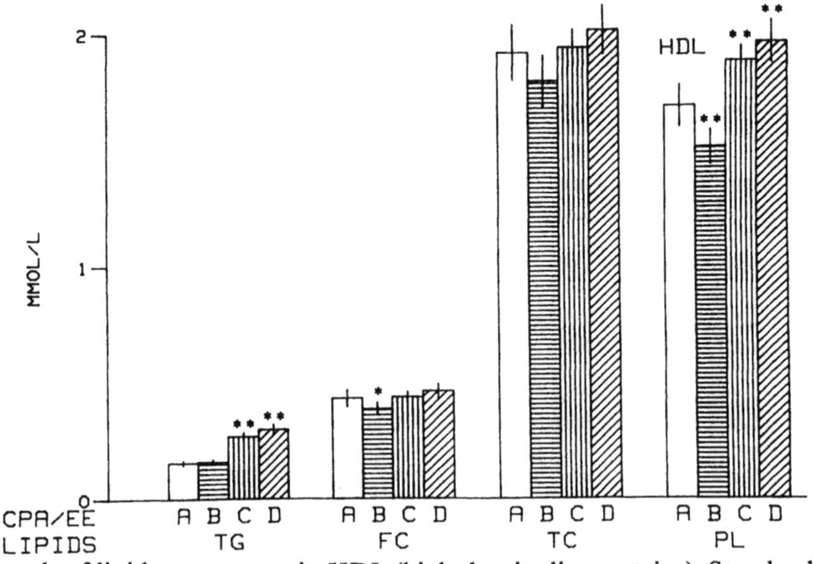

Fig. 3 Levels of lipid components in HDL (high-density lipoproteins). See also legend to figure 2.

HDL-lipids: When administered alone, 2 mg cyproterone acetate induced a decrease in FC ($p < 0.05$) and PL ($p < 0.01$). When 2 mg cyproterone acetate + 35 μg ethinyl estradiol were used, there was an increase in TG and PL ($p < 0.01$). These latter changes were seen also with 2 mg cyproterone acetate + 50 μg ethinyl estradiol (fig. 3).

Discussion

In this study the cyproterone acetate/ethinyl estradiol combinations induced a substantial increase of TG, both in serum and in all lipoprotein fractions. This influence is an almost constant finding after administration of alkylated estrogens (ethinyl estradiol or mestranol), alone or in "estrogen dominated" oral contraceptives [5, 1, 10]. Although increased TG-levels in serum and in the VLDL fraction is a risk factor for cardiovascular disease (CVD), at least in elderly women [8, 6], more attention has been directed toward influences on the HDL and LDL fractions in this context.

Cyproterone acetate is a 17-hydroxyprogesterone derivative. Previous studies have shown that steroids derived from 17-hydroxyprogesterone have less antiestrogenic effects than do 19-nortestosterone derivatives. In accordance with these findings, cyproterone acetate did not counteract the typical effects on serum lipids induced by ethinyl estradiol to any major extent.

The use of an oral contraceptive with predominantly estrogenic effects to ameliorate clinical expressions of hyperandrogenism such as acne, seborrhoea and hirsutism, induces an increase in SHBG. This increase exerts its well-documented therapeutic effects through an increased binding and inactivation of the androgens. With oral contraceptives, induction of increased SHBG-levels appears to be accompanied by concomitant elevations of the serum-TG [11].

In women on oral contraceptives increased serum and VLDL TG levels may occur concomitantly with increased HDL-CH levels. This may be regarded as a "beneficial" effect with respect to risk of cardiovascular disease. It cannot be said with certainity whether this concomitant increase in VLDL and HDL has any significance for risk of cardiovascular disease. However, it is hardly a physiological influence as there tends to be an inverse relationship between VLDL and HDL in non-pharmacological conditions [14, 3].

Does this increase in serum and VLDL-TG have any clinical implications? For the vast majority of young women in need of antiandrogen treatment, the increase in serum and VLDL-TG can probably be looked upon with equanimity.

Women with hirsutism as part of the polycystic ovary syndrome (PCO), however, should probably receive special attention. These women are more obese and have higher blood pressure. Furthermore, two recent studies demonstrate that they also have substantially higher serum and VLDL TG-levels than regularly menstruating women [12, 17]. Cullberg et al. [2] have shown that "estrogen dominated" oral contraceptives further increase these elevated TG-levels in PCO women. Consequently, the increase in TG caused by exogenous sex steroids, may further deteriorate an already somewhat adverse situation with respect to atherogenic risk factors. It is therefore advisable to monitor serum TG in these women before and during treatment, at least in those over thirty years of age and those intending to use the antiandrogenic preparation for several years.

Cyproterone acetate administered alone and in this low dose had little influence on lipoprotein lipids. There was a small decrease in HDL-Pl, which probably had no biological significance.

Conclusion

For the vast majority of women in need of antiandrogen treatment the effects on TG-metabolism induced by these ethinyl estradiol/cyproterone acetate combinations should be looked upon with equanimity. A few patients may, however, need special attention.

Acknowledgements
Thanks are due to Ms Lena Cederlund, Ms Görel Gundersen and Ms Margareta Medberg for technical assistance and to Ms Kerstin Meyer for secretarial help. The kind supply of cyproterone acetate and ethinyl estradiol (Schering AG, Berlin, West Germany) is acknowledged.

This work was supported by a grant from Göteborgs Läkaresällskap.

References

[1] Crona, N., G. Silfverstolpe, G. Samsioe: Does progestogen reduction in oral contraception parallel reduced lipid metabolic effects? Acta Obstet. Gynecol. Scand. Suppl. **105** (1982) 41—44.

[2] Cullberg, G., L. Hamberger, L-Å. Mattsson et al.: Lipid metabolic studies in women with a polycystic ovary syndrome during treatment with a low dose desogestrel-ethinylestradiol combination. Acta Obstet. Gynecol. Scand. **64** (1985) 203—207.

[3] Davis, C. E., D. Gordon, J. la Rosa et al.: Correlations of plasma high-density lipoprotein cholesterol levels with other plasma lipid and lipoprotein concentrations. Circulation 62, Suppl. **IV** (1980) 24—30.

[4] Furman, R. H., P. Alaupovic, R. P. Howard: Effects of androgens and estrogens on serum lipids and the composition and concentration of serum lipoproteins in normolipemic and hyperlipidemic states. Progr. Biochem. Pharmacol. **2** (1967) 215—249.

[5] Goldzieher, J. W., C. B. Chenault, A. de la Pena et al.: Comparative studies of the ethinyl estrogens used in oral contraceptives. VII Effects with and without progestational agents on ultracentrifugally fractionated plasma lipoproteins in humans, baboons and beagles. Fertil. Steril. **30** (1978) 522—533.
[6] Gordon, T., W. P. Castelli, M. C. Hjortland et al.: High density lipoprotein as a protective factor against coronary heart disease. Am. J. Med **62** (1977) 707—714.
[7] Hirvonen, E., M. Mälkönen, V. Manninen: Effects of different progestogens on lipoproteins during postmenopausal replacement therapy. N. Engl. J. Med. **304** (1981) 560—563.
[8] Johansson, S. et al.: Serum apolipoproteins and alphalipoprotein cholesterol levels in relation to acute myocardial infarction and its established risk factors in women. Diss. University of Göteborg, Sweden. (1983).
[9] Kay, C. R.: Progestogens and arterial disease—evidence from the Royal College of General Practitioners' study. Am. J. Obstet. Gynecol. **142** (1980) 762—765.
[10] Knopp, R. et al.: Oral contraceptive and postmenopausal estrogen effects on lipoprotein triglyceride and cholesterol in an adult female population: relationship to estrogen and progestin potency. J. Clin. Endocrinol. Metabol. **53** (1981) 1123—1132.
[11] Larsson-Cohn, U., L. Fåhraeus, L. Wallentin et al.: Lipoprotein changes may be minimized by proper composition of a combined oral contraceptive. Fertil. Steril. **35** (1981) 172—179.
[12] Mattsson, L-Å., G. Cullberg, L. Hamberger et al.: Lipid metabolism in women with polycystic ovary syndrome: possible implications for an increased risk of coronary heart disease. Fertil. Steril. **42** (1984) 579—584.
[13] Meade, W., G. Greenberg, S. G. Thompson: Progestogens and cardiovascular reactions associated with oral contraceptives and a comparison of the safety of 50- and 30-μg oestrogen preparations. Br. Med. J. **280** (1980) 1157—1161.
[14] Schaeffer, E. J., D. W. Andersson, H. B. Brewer et al.: Plasma-triglycerides in regulation of HDL-cholesterol levels. Lancet **2** (1978) 391—392.
[15] Silfverstolpe, G., A. Gustavsson, G. Samsioe et al.: Lipid metabolic studies in oophorectomized women. Effects of three different progestogens. Acta Obstet. Gynecol. Scand. Suppl. **88** (1979) 89—95.
[16] Walton, K. W., P. J. Scott, P. W. Dykes et al.: The significance of alterations in serum lipids in thyroid dysfunction. II. Alterations of the metabolism and turnover of ^{131}-I-low density lipoproteins in hypothyroidism and thyrotoxicosis. Clin. Sci. **29** (1965) 217—238.
[17] Wild, R. A., P. C. Painter, P. B. Coulson et al.: Lipoprotein lipid concentrations and cardiovascular risk in women with polycystic ovary syndrome. J. Clin. Endocrinol. Metabol. **61** (1985) 946—951.
[18] Witztum, J., G. Schonfelt: High density lipoproteins. Diab. **28** (1979) 326—336.

Clinical, metabolic and endocrine effects of long term use of a cyproterone acetate and ethinyl estradiol combination in hyperandrogenized women

U. J. Gaspard, J. Bonnivert, P. Emonts, D. Gillain, R. Lambotte

Introduction

It has been well established in numerous studies over the past ten years or more that the reverse sequential combination of high doses (50 to 100 mg) of cyproterone acetate, a 17-OH progesterone derived progestin with antiandrogen properties, and 50 mcg ethinyl estradiol is very effective in the long-term treatment (6 to 12 months and more) of hirsutism [7, 9] and of other signs of androgenization such as alopecia, seborrhea and acne. These latter symptoms are also rapidly and effectively improved by lower doses of cyproterone acetate (2 mg) combined with 50 mcg of ethinyl estradiol or Diane® [8, 2]. However, in spite of excellent cycle control, the lack of antiestrogenic activity of cyproterone acetate and the relatively large amount of ethinyl estradiol contained in this preparation can cause estrogen-related side-effects such as breast tension and weight increase. An interesting and unexpected observation with Diane® is that mild to moderate hirsutism is distinctly improved in almost 50% of the cases in spite of the small amount of antiandrogen in this preparation [8, 2]. As cyproterone acetate, which is devoid of androgenic effects, is associated with fewer metabolic adverse effects than other progestins such as those derived from 19 nortestosterone, it was tempting to use it in larger amounts than in Diane® and to combine it with a low-dose of ethinyl estradiol. We accordingly used a preparation containing cyproterone acetate 5 mg and ethinyl estradiol 35 mcg in order to obtain a potentially more effective antiandrogen action with less estrogen dominance than in the former combination. We tested this preparation for a period of 18 months in a straight open study of 29 female patients presenting successively with acne and/or hirsutism and seborrhea in order to verify its clinical effectiveness, and its effects on hormones, lipids and liver function tests.

Methods

a) Subjects

The 29 female patients investigated had a mean age of 23.7 yrs ± 1.32 (mean + SEM) and the following clinical characteristics : height 163 ± 1.25 cm, weight 58.9 ± 1.99 kg, systolic blood pressure 121 ± 2.1 mmHg, and diastolic blood pressure 73 ± 1.2 mmHg. Cycles were irregular with an oligomenorrheic trend and were associated with acne in 72% of the subjects, hirsutism in 69% and seborrhea in 36% (frequently combined). Moreover, dysmenorrhea was present in 45% and a mild to moderate premenstrual tension syndrome was recorded in 48% of the subjects. All patients underwent a complete gynecological examination and those with contra-indications to oral contraceptive use were excluded from the study. A dermatological evaluation of acne, seborrhea, and hirsutism was made before treatment and after 6, 12, and 18 months of use of the test preparation. Usual clinical criteria were used to determine the dermatological status of seborrhea and acne. Lesions were graded as follows: 1 = mild, 2 = moderate, 3 = severe. Hirsutism was evaluated according to the classification proposed by Abraham et al. [1]. The patients were examined by the same investigator on each occasion.

After clinical evaluation, selection, and cessation of oral contraceptive or other sex steroid use for at least two cycles, a blood specimen was drawn seven days before presumed menstruation during a pre-treatment spontaneous cycle.

The test preparation containing 5 mg cyproterone acetate (CPA) and 35 mcg ethinyl estradiol (EE) was then administered daily from day 1 of the first treatment cycle for 21 successive days and followed by a drug-free interval of 7 days. This treatment was repeated for a period of 18 months. Clinical and biologic evaluations were again performed during the last 3 days of treatment in cycles 6, 12, and 18.

b) Biologic assays

Hormone, lipid, and hepatic function tests were carried out using specific assays previously described [3, 5, 2].

Results

1. General clinical assessment

The test preparation was well tolerated, and remarkably few subjective or objective complaints were recorded (tab. 1). There were especially few complaints

Table 1 Subjective complaints of the patients before and during treatment with cyproterone acetate and ethinyl estradiol (in percent of cases)

Complaint	Pre-treatment	6 months	12 months	18 months
Nervousness	6	3	3	0
Depression	0	3	0	0
Headache	15	6	0	3
Nausea	0	0	0	0
Loss of libido	0	0	0	3
Chloasma	0	3	3	3
Water retention	6	3	0	3
Breast pain	9	6	15	0

about breast tension and water retention. No pregnancy was recorded during the study. Cycle control was excellent and characterised by a progressive shortening of the cycle from a mean pre-treatment length of 37.4 days to a normal mean cycle length of 27.5 days and a mean delay between cessation of treatment and the first day of the following menstruation of 4.8 days. Chi square analyses revealed a significant ($P < 0.01$) decrease in dysmenorrhea and premenstrual tension (fig. 1). Cumulated frequencies of spotting and breakthrough bleeding either before or during treatment were observed in fewer than 5% of the cycles studied. No patient dropped out of the study because of reasons related to the drug. Weight changes were slight: a non-significant mean of 500 gm weight increase was recorded after 18 months of treatment. Blood pressure remained unchanged.

2. Symptoms of androgenization

Seborrhea regressed completely in 9 out of 10 patients after only 3 to 6 months of treatment (fig. 1). Acne disappeared completely in 81% of the patients and was partially improved in the remaining 19%. Improvement was already discernible at 3—6 months and increased slightly thereafter until the end of the treatment period.

Hirsutism showed a marked improvement in 14 out 20 patients (70%). This improvement proceeded more slowly than the acne improvement but remained continuous until the 18th month of therapy. Six patients (30%) were either slightly or not improved. For each of these symptoms, and for each localization (face, chest, shoulders, abdomen, limbs . . .) chi square analysis revealed a significant decrease ($p < 0.01$) during treatment.

3. Laboratory findings

— **Lipids:** Total serum triglyceride concentrations increased non-significantly for the first 12 months of treatment. At 18 months, a 50% increase over basal

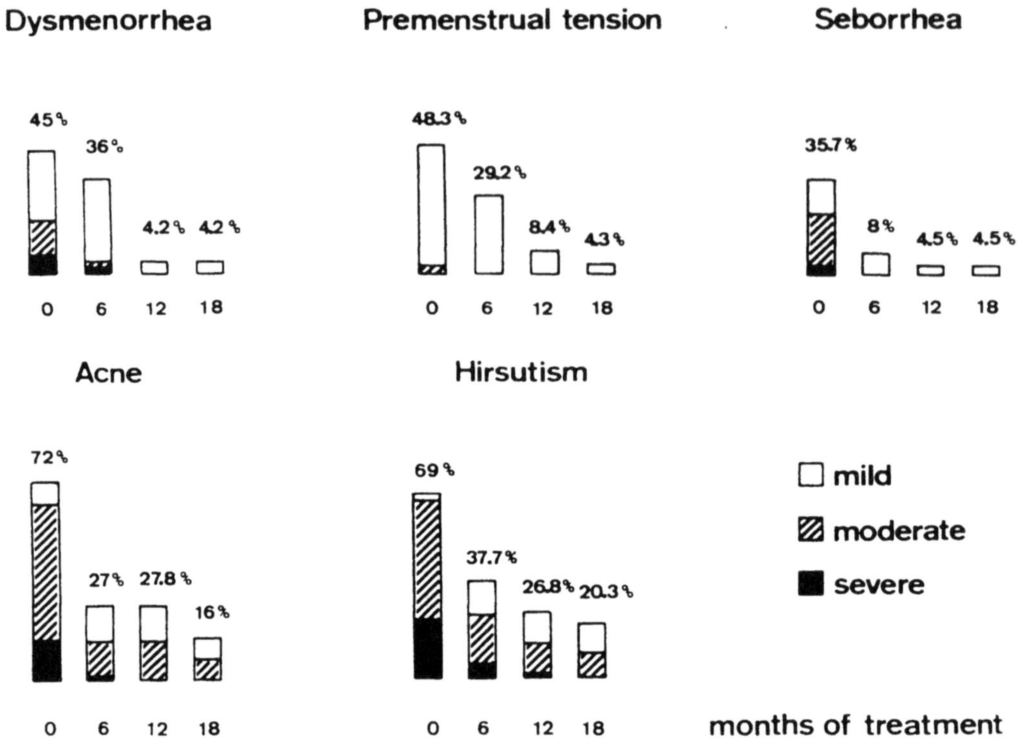

Fig. 1 Therapeutic effectiveness of a preparation containing 5 mg cyproterone acetate combined with 35 mcg ethinyl estradiol in 29 hyperandrogenized women.

levels was statistically significant (tab. 2). Although total cholesterol concentrations increased moderately (17%), this increase was not significant. HDL-cholesterol levels were unchanged during the whole study.

— **Hepatic tests:** No change in the results of hepatic function tests was recorded at any time in this study.

— **Hormone levels:** Pre-treatment levels of estradiol and estrone were in the normal range for our laboratory values. Progesterone levels were low, and some androgen levels were at the upper limit of our normal range, particularly the total and free testosterone concentration levels. After 18 months of use of the preparation under study, the mean level of estradiol (E_2) was 19%, estrone (E_1) 28%, progesterone (P) 6%, total testosterone (T) 57%, free testosterone 23%, dihydrotestosterone (DHT) 100%, dehydroepiandrosterone sulfate (DS) 70%, androstenedione (A) 58%, sex hormone binding globulin (SHBG) 312%, and cortisol 206% of basal pre-treatment levels respectively. Most of these changes were statistically significant (tab. 2).

Table 2 Serum levels of biologic parameters before and during treatment with cyproterone acetate and ethinyl estradiol in 29 female patients

		Pre-treatment (1)	6 months (2)	12 months (3)	18 months (4)	P
LIPIDS						
Triglycerides	mg/dl	82.7 ± 4.0	102.2 ± 7.5	103.2 ± 3.4	128.1 ± 4.0	1,2 vs 4 0.024
Total cholesterol	mg/dl	163.8 ± 16.9	147.4 ± 15.0	196.1 ± 9.3	191.1 ± 30.0	NS
HDL-cholesterol	mg/dl	61.4 ± 9.3	56.0 ± 3.9	66.2 ± 1.6	58.1 ± 6.6	NS
HEPATIC TESTS						
Total bilirubin	mg/l	6.9 ± 1.4	4.9 ± 0.9	4.2 ± 0.9	4.3 ± 0.7	NS
Conjugated bilirubin	mg/l	1.5 ± 0.1	1.4 ± 0.2	1.4 ± 0.1	1.3 ± 0.1	NS
Alkaline Phosphatase	IU/l	59.1 ± 3.6	68.1 ± 7.1	63.5 ± 7.0	52.0 ± 3.5	NS
SGOT	IU/l	20.2 ± 1.7	23.5 ± 3.3	16.3 ± 1.1	17.3 ± 1.0	NS
SGPT	IU/l	19.5 ± 2.3	20.6 ± 2.5	17.4 ± 2.6	17.2 ± 2.4	NS
HORMONES						
Estradiol	pg/ml	124 ± 21	40 ± 19	32 ± 6	23 ± 6	1 vs 2,3,4 0.002
Estrone	pg/ml	63 ± 8	53 ± 15	42 ± 8	18 ± 2	1 vs 4 0.005
Progesterone	ng/ml	3.74 ± 1.29	0.21 ± 0.05	0.384 ± 0.07	0.258 ± 0.03	1 vs 2,3,4 0.005
Total testosterone	pg/ml	523 ± 40	396 ± 50	347 ± 22	298 ± 49	1,2 vs 4 0.01
Free testosterone	pg/ml	6.41 ± 0.96	3.40 ± 0.96	2.35 ± 0.53	1.46 ± 0.31	1 vs 3,4 0.003
SHBG	nMol/l	78 ± 10	224 ± 31	263 ± 41	242 ± 55	1 vs 2,3,4 0.008
Dihydrotestosterone	pg/ml	240 ± 27	223 ± 55	243 ± 47	240 ± 86	NS
Dehydroepiandrosterone sulfate	ng/ml	2501 ± 243	1890 ± 281	1868 ± 297	1753 ± 319	1 vs 4 0.05
Δ_4-androstenedione	pg/ml	2112 ± 171	1236 ± 130	1520 ± 245	1580 ± 305	1 vs 2,3,4 0.05
Cortisol	ng/ml	131 ± 23	262 ± 35	231 ± 37	271 ± 17	1 vs 2,3,4 0.01

Discussion

An objective and subjective general clinical assessment of the long-term tolerance of this intermediate to low dose cyproterone acetate (5 mg) and low-dose ethinyl estradiol (35 mcg) preparation shows a very low level of complaints and side-effects. This indicates an interesting clinical balance of this preparation; it is apparently devoid of the estrogenic side effects of the Diane® containing 50 mcg ethinyl estradiol [8, 2]. This is also reflected in a marked decrease in the frequency of dysmenorrhea and premenstrual tension which also reflects a lack of clinical estrogen dominance in the preparation under study.

With both preparations, the one containing 5 mg cyproterone acetate and the one containing 2 mg cyproterone acetate, cycle control is excellent and contraceptive effectiveness is optimal. As expected, acne and seborrhea regress quickly and completely in 80% and 90% of the subjects treated, respectively, while the remaining 20% and 10% are partially improved. This result is comparable to the one repeatedly observed with either high-dose or low-dose combinations of cyproterone acetate and ethinyl estradiol [7, 8, 2, 6, and review in 4]. The observation of a rather high level of improvement of hirsutism with the preparation under study (5 mg cyproterone acetate) is particularly interesting. In fact, although before treatment 1 patient displayed a mild hirsutism, 13 moderate hirsutism, and 6 severe hirsutism, by the end of the treatment period in 14 cases (70%) excess hair had completely regressed, in 3 patients only mild hirsutism was present and in 3 moderate hirsutism. Although this series is limited, it seems to compare favorably with improvement rates in mild to moderate cases of hirsutism submitted to Diane® treatment reported earlier [8, 2].

Although the preparation studied (cyproterone acetate 5 mg and ethinyl estradiol 35 mcg) demonstrates weaker estrogenic effects than does Diane® (cyproterone acetate 2 mg and ethinyl estradiol 50 mcg), the difference at metabolic end points is less obvious: both preparations behave in a slightly estrogenic manner and their long-term use is accordingly associated with a moderate increase in triglycerides and total cholesterol with unchanged levels of HDL-cholesterol. These results are in agreement with other studies [2, 10] and underline the lack of any androgenic/antiestrogenic effect of preparations containing cyproterone acetate and ethinyl estradiol, as opposed to the effects of other oral contraceptive combinations.

As relates to serum hormone levels, the use of the preparation cyproterone acetate 5 mg and ethinyl estradiol 35 mcg is associated with an effective inhibition of gonadal function which is strictly comparable to the endocrine effects of either Diane® (cyproterone acetate 2 mg and ethinyl estradiol 50 mcg) [2, 4] or the high-dose reverse sequential preparation [9]. This is reflected by low levels of E_2 and E_1 during the whole period of treatment, low anovulatory levels of P, low levels of A and total T, and particularly depressed levels of free T. On the other hand, due to the estrogenic action of the preparation studied, SHBG and transcortin are distinctly increased. This explains the only transiently decreased levels of DHT (which binds with very high affinity to SHBG) and the increased levels of cortisol. The slightly decreased levels of DS may be partly related to a direct inhibitory effect of this preparation on the adrenals.

Conclusion

In conclusion, clinically the long-term use (18 months) of a preparation containing 5 mg cyproterone acetate and 35 mcg ethinyl estradiol is subjectively and objectively well tolerated. No sign of estrogen dominance appears. It effectively improves not only acne and seborrhea, but also hirsutism in spite of its rather low content of cyproterone acetate. It additionally inhibits gonadal function and decreases circulating androgen levels. From a metabolic viewpoint, it still behaves as a slightly estrogen-dominant preparation, as indicated by a moderate increase in triglyceride levels and a more distinct increase in SHBG. Total and HDL-cholesterol levels are not significantly altered. This preparation is characterized by a good balance of clinical and metabolic effects and is therefore particularly interesting for long-term use in the treatment of women with androgenization symptoms.

Acknowledgments
We wish to thank Mrs. A. M. Verly-Smolnik for excellent secretarial assistance.

References

[1] Abraham, G. E., G. B. Maroulis, J. E. Buster et al.: Effect of dexamethazone on serum cortisol and androgen levels in hirsute patients. Obstet. Gynecol. **47** (1976) 395—402.
[2] Gaspard, U. J., M. A. Romus, M. Soyeur-Broux et al.: Clinical, endocrinological, and metabolic evaluation of women treated for acne by a combination of cyproterone acetate and ethinylestradiol (Diane®). In: Vokaer, R., D. Fanta (eds.): Combined antiandrogen-estrogen therapy in dermatology, pp. 75—93. Excerpta Medica, Amsterdam 1981.
[3] Gaspard, U. J., M. A. Romus, D. Gillain et al.: Plasma hormone levels in women receiving new oral contraceptives containing ethinyl estradiol plus levonorgestrel or desogestrel. Contraception **27** (1983) 577—590.
[4] Gaspard, U. J.: Role of antiandrogens in the treatment of acne. In: Mahesh, V. B., R. B. Greenblatt (eds.): Hirsutism and Virilism, pp. 369—394. Wright-PSG, Boston 1983.
[5] Gaspard, U. J., J. Buret, D. Gillain et al.: Serum lipid and lipoprotein changes induced by new oral contraceptives containing ethinyl estradiol plus levonorgestrel or desogestrel. Contraception **31** (1985) 395—408.

[6] Greenwood, R., L. Brummitt, B. Burke et al.: Acne: double blind clinical and laboratory trial of tetracycline, oestrogen-cyproterone acetate, and combined treatment. Br. Med. J. **291** (1985) 1231—1235.
[7] Hammerstein, J., J. Meckies, I. Leo-Rossberg et al.: Use of cyproterone acetate in the treatment of acne, hirsutism and virilism. J. Ster. Biochem. **6** (1975) 827—836.
[8] Moltz, L., J. Meckies, J. Hammerstein: Die Kontrazeptive Betreuung androgenisierter Frauen mit einem niedrig dosierten cyproteron acetat-haltigen Einphasenpräparat. Dtsch. Med. Wschr. **104** (1979) 1376—1382.
[9] Rubens, R.: Androgen levels during cyproterone acetate and ethinylestradiol treatment of hirsutism. Clin. Endocr. (Oxf) **20** (1984) 313—325.
[10] Tikkanen, M. J., T. Kuusi, E. A. Nikkilä et al.: Absence of lipoprotein changes during treatment with cyproterone acetate. Arch. Gynec. **237** (1985) 130 A.

Cyproterone acetate versus levonorgestrel combined with ethinyl estradiol in the treatment of acne: results of a multi-center study

L. Carlborg

Introduction

Although acne is not an endocrine disease, it is clearly dependent upon sex steroids. The primary site of the disease is the infrainfundibulum of the sebaceous glands located where there are glands with a rudimentary hair follicle, that is on the face, on the back, and on the chest. Androgens increase cell proliferation in the infrainfundibulum. These cells slough off easily and may form a plug and thus cause retention of sebum. The bacteria which is always in sebaceous glands then cleave the sebum into fatty acids. Through small ruptures of the gland wall, fatty acids can then protrude into the surrounding area. Leucocytes are attracted and the well-known acne lesion is formed. Estrogens, in contrast, reduce the cell proliferation of the infrainfundibulum.

Some clinical facts will elucidate the importance of androgens. Hypogonadel males are free from acne but when they receive substitution treatment with androgens, it may develop. No acne is found in eunuchs. Acne is not found in adolescent girls until they get their menarche or adrenarche when androgens are formed. In women, acne often develops in cases of androgenetic disturbances such as the polycystic ovary (PCO) syndrome or andrenal over-activity. Increased plasma androgen levels or indirect signs of higher androgen turnover in women with acne as compared to healthy women have been demonstrated [8]. The most active androgen is dihydro-testosterone which acts directly on the cell nucleus. In some patients there is an increased conversion of low-activity androgens into testosterone or dihydro-testosterone because of an increased amount of 5-α-reductase in the skin [9]. In cases of an overproduction of androgens from the ovary, oral contraceptives have often been used to inactivate the ovary. Most of the gestagens used in oral contraceptives belong to the 19-nortestosterone group and may thus have some intrinsic androgen activity. They may also replace testosterone from the sexhormone binding globulin which thus becomes biologically available. Many acne patients deteriorate when using oral contraceptives [6]. In cases in which the androgen overproduction is of adrenal origin, dexamethasone suppression is sometimes used.

Regardless of the origin of the androgen causing acne, it is logical to use antiandrogens which act directly on the target cell by blocking the receptor site. Many antiandrogens belong to the 17-OH progesterone group. The most active compound known is cyproterone acetate (CPA). It is also a strong gestagen. Numerous studies have shown that when combined with ethinyl estradiol (2 mg cyproterone acetate and 50 microgram ethinyl estradiol: Diane®), this substance is extremely useful in the treatment of acne in women [3, 4, 5].

Although the effect of Diane® on acne is well documented, objective studies using quantitative methods are still needed. Comparison with a suitable oral contraceptive [5, 1] should be made and an estimation of acne should be made by a dermatologist.

Material and methods

The present study was designed as a cooperation between gynecologists and dermatologists at 8 centres in Sweden. Women suffering from acne who were over 15 years of age and had no contraindications to the use of oral contraceptives were enrolled in the study. The observation period was 6 months and the study design was double-blind. The patients were 160 volunteers (most of them aged 20—29 years) who were treated from autumn to spring so as to exclude the possible beneficial effect of the sun on acne. The consent of all patients was gained and the study was accepted by the Swedish National Board of Health and Welfare and the Ethical Committees.

Three treatment preparations were subject to study: Diane® (see above), Diane-35® with a dose of only 35 mcg ethinyl estradiol and Neovletta (150 mcg levonorgestrel and 30 mcg ethinyl estradiol) as the reference preparation.

The *gynecologist* collected data on spontaneous menstrual bleeding pattern, previous use of contraceptives, and gynecologic health. Six 21-day packages of one of the three test preparations were distributed at random to each patient. Control visits were made after 2 and after 6 cycles.

The *dermatologist* counted the number of acne lesions (sum of pustules, papules, cysts, and nodules) in the face and on the cheeks. Other locations of acne were disregarded. A minimum of 8 was required [1, 6] for inclusion in the study. No specific treatment of acne was allowed 4 weeks prior to treatment or during the study. Controls were made after 4 and 6 cycles.

The gynecologist, dermatologist, and patient each subjectively evaluated the treatment in terms of good, moderate, or poor at the last check-up.

At the start of the trial the absolute number of acne lesions varied considerably from one patient to another: it varied between 8 and 100 with a majority falling in the range of 12—23 lesions. Therefore, treatment data had to be transformed to per cent change from start value. At least 8 lesions were required for inclusion in the study. Since data within a treatment group were statistically not normally distributed, non-parametric statistical methods were used (Kruskal-Wallis and Wilcoxon). When appropriate, the Chi square test and / or Tukey's studentized range test were used. All data were processed by computer.

Results

Of the 160 volunteers who entered the study, 136 were suitable for inclusion in the computer program. Those who did not fulfill inclusion criteria, interrupted treatment because of worsening or side effects, stopped participation or for whom protocols were incomplete were excluded. These drop-outs were evenly distributed in the three treatment groups which became of about the same size. All groups were homogenous with regard to their gynecological/obstetrical history and with regard to the acne disease which, on the average, had persisted for over nine years. Many had been treated earlier with other methods but with only poor results.

Dermatological evaluation

After four cycles Diane® and Diane-35® resulted in a similar reduction of acne to about 55% of the baseline value. Neovletta resulted in an average reduction of only 27%. These results were statistically different at $P<0.05$ (tab. 1).

After six cycles, Diane® and Diane-35® produced a reduction of about 70% but Neovletta produced only half of this improvement, a statistically signifi-

Table 1 Mean (± SD) per cent reduction of facial acne after 4 months of treatment. Diane and Diane 35 were found to be significantly more effective than Neovletta at $p < 0.05$ (Wilcoxon Rank Sum Test)

Test preparation	n	Reduction % ± SD
Diane	46	51 ± 52
Diane-35	45	61 ± 31
Neovletta	37	27 ± 52

Table 2 Mean (± SD) per cent reduction of facial acne after 6 months of treatment. Diane and Diane 35 were found to be significantly more effective than Neovletta at $p < 0.0001$ (Wilcoxon Rank Sum Test)

Test preparation	n	Reduction % ± SD
Diane	45	70 ± 36
Diane-35	44	72 ± 27
Neovletta	36	35 ± 60

cant difference at $P<0.0001$ (tab. 2). In the sixth cycle more than 60% of the patients in the Diane® and Diane-35® groups had at least 75% reduction of acne compared to only 26% in the Neovletta group (tab. 3). Only 4% in the Diane® and the Diane-35® groups and 18% in the Neovletta group deteriorated.

Table 3 Per cent of patients within a treatment group who experienced at least 75% reduction of facial acne and per cent patients who experienced no change or deterioration after 6 months of treatment

Test preparation	n	≧ 75% reduction	no change or worse
Diane	45	66	4.3
Diane-35	44	61	4.5
Neovletta	36	26	17.8

The subjective assessments made by the gynecologist, dermatologist, and patient were, on the average, similar and showed with statistical significance that Diane® and Diane-35® were superior to Neovletta for the treatment of acne (tab. 4).

Table 4 Average subjective assessments of the results of the treatment regimens in cycle 6. Score: 1 = good, 2 = moderate, 3 = poor. Diane and Diane 35 were unanimously judged to be better than Neovletta at $p < 0.001$ (Wilcoxon/Kruskall-Wallis Test).

Test preparation	n	Mean score given by gynecologist	dermatologist	patient
Diane	45	1.36	1.42	1.38
Diane-35	44	1.23	1.49	1.41
Neovletta	36	1.75	2.00	2.03

Gynecological evaluation

No pregnancy occurred in any group, thus indicating that all products tested are good contraceptives. Cycle length as well as the amount of bleeding was usually unaffected by all three test preparations. Patients with previous excessive bleedings tended to achieve a reduced flow using any of the preparations. Absence of withdrawal bleeding never occurred after Diane® or Daine-35®, but did occur in 1 to 2 cycles regularly among 36 users of Neovletta. Spotting and breakthrough bleeding occurred as expected in the first cycles and decreased with time. No important difference was seen among the preparations. Body weight and blood pressure remained almost unaffected.

Side effects

Emphasis was put on side effects spontaneously reported by the patient but some questioning was also made by the gynecologist. In the first cycles nausea was more common in the Diane® group but it decreased by the sixth cycle. Breast tension was slightly more common in the Diane® group than in the Neovletta group. Six women on Neovletta, 6 women on Diane®, and five women on Diane-35® discontinued use due to side effects. Varicose complaints, headache, nervousness, chloasma, edema, depression, and decreased libido were infrequent and similarly present in all groups. In summary, it can be concluded that all side effects were of minor seriousness and comparable to those shown to be associated with the use of other oral contraceptives [2].

Discussion

This study shows that Diane® and Diane-35® are equally highly effective in the treatment of acne and that both are significantly better than a "regular" oral contraceptive (Neovletta®). The study also confirms earlier observations that oral contraceptives may cure acne in some patients. Unfortunately, some get worse and we do not know how to select these from the beginning. The reduction of the estrogen dose in Diane-35® not only produced an excellent bleeding pattern but also appeared to reduce the rate of occurence and severity of some of the side effects believed to be caused by the estrogen component.

It has been pointed out that the patient's own evaluation of an acne treatment should have a large impact on the total evaluation as the disease is of great cosmetic importance. This study clearly shows that there is a satisfactory agreement between the patient's subjective evaluation and the objectively measured data. Therefore, other studies on Diane® treatment using subjective methods are probably reliable.

The reduction of ethinyl estradiol from 50 mcg in Diane® to 35 mcg in Diane-35® appears to be successful. The excellent effect on acne is maintained and, in addition, an excellent bleeding pattern and a reduction of "estrogenic" side effects are achieved. It is suggested as the method of choice for women with acne who accept an oral contraceptive.

References

[1] Allen, B. S., G. Smith: Various parameters for grading acne vulgaris. Arch. Dermatol. **118** (1982) 23.
[2] Bye, P.: Analysis of a multicenter trial of a new low-dose oral contraceptive in Great Britain. Acta. Obstet. Gynecol. Scand. Suppl. **54** (1976) 61—66.
[3] Carlborg, L., S. Rosengren: Antiandrogen treatment of women with acne tarda. Curr. Ther. Res. **31** (1982) 740—745.
[4] Fanta, D.: Acne. Springer. Wien—New York 1978.
[5] Lachnit-Fixson, U., J. Kaufmann: Zur Beeinflussung von Androgenisierungserscheinungen. Med. Klin. **72** (1977) 1922—1926.
[6] Lachnit-Fixson, U.: The development and evaluation of an ovulation inhibito (Diane) containing an antiandrogen. Acta. Obstet. Gynecol. Scand. Suppl. **88** (1979) 33—42.
[7] Lidén, S. et al.: Clinical Evaluation in Acne. Acta. Dermatovenerol. (Stockholm) Suppl. **89** (1980).
[8] Odlind, V., K. Carlström, G. Michaelsson et al.: Plasma androgenic activity in women with acne vulgaris and in healthy girls before, during and after puberty. Clin. Endocrinol. **16** (1982) 243—249.
[9] Sansone, G., R. M. Reisner: Differential rates of conversion of testosterone to dihydrotestosterone in acne and in normal human skin—A possible pathogenic factor in acne. J. Invest. Dermatol. **56** (1971) 366.

Acknowledgement
The following gynecologists and dermatologists participated in this multi-center study:

Falun: Börje Lindström, Staffan Nilsson, Eva-Brita Strålin.

Göteborg: Kjell Hersle, Per Olof Janson, Håkan Mobacken, Lars Nilsson.

Halmstad: Lars Carlborg, Kerstin Olsson.

Malmö: Bertil Casslén, Eva Jepson, Lars Svanberg.

Stockholm: Erik Borglund, Bengt-Åke Lindhe, Anna-Kristina von Uexküll, Göran Wennersten.

Umeå: Ove Bäck, Mats Göran Damberg, Bo von Schoultz.

Uppsala: Annika Bergkvist-Karlsson, Viveca Odlind.

The author also wants to express his gratitude to:

Prof Gösta Hagerman and Prof Sture Lidén for their valuable advice in dermatological questions. The computer programs and the statistical evaluations were kindly performed by Ass Prof Mats Ehrnebo, Galenus AB, Uppsala. This study was supported by Schering AG, Federal Republic of Germany and Schering Nordiska AB, Sweden.

Comparison of Diane-35® with Neo-Eunomin® from the dermatological viewpoint

F. Nürnberger

Introduction

Acne vulgaris is a chronic inflammatory disorder of the pilo-sebaceous follicles, mostly of the face, back, chest and shoulders [2]. The *causal pathogenesis of acne* is multifactorial ("Causation mosaic"): it involves follicles, sebum, bacteria, hormones, heredity, and the immune system. If one factor of the "mosaic" is missing, e. g., the hormones (androgenes), no acne will occur. No acne occurs in castrated males.

1. Follicles: There are three types of facial follicles: Vellus follicles, sebaceous follicles, and terminal beard hair follicles. Especially the sebaceous follicles with their large sebum glands are the target organ for acne. In acne patients these sebaceous follicles have probably a genetically determined (?) enhanced propensity for hyperkeratosis, comedo formation in the infrainfundibulum, and for follicular and peri-follicular inflammation.

2. Sebum (Seborrhoea): Sebum is a mixture of glyceride and fatty acids (65%), sqalene (10%) and wax esters (25%). Acne patients usually have seborrhoea, i. e., sebum production and skin surface lipids are enhanced [1].

Seborrhoea, however, can also be found without acne in rosacea, gram-negative folliculitis, seborrheic dermatitis, and Parkinson-Syndrome. Bacterial lipases split off free fatty acids from di- and triglycerides (see below).

3. Bacteria: Deeper parts of the sebaceous follicles are colonized by Propionibacterium acnes and Propionibacterium granulosum (= Corynebacterium acnes, types 1 and 2). Bacterial ectolipases split sebum triglycerides into glycerin and free fatty acids. The free fatty acids cause infundibular hyperkeratosis, comedones, follicular and peri-follicular inflammation. Bacterial products of P. acnes (mucopolysaccharides, enzymes, prostaglandin-like substances in the lipid fraction of P. acnes) act as mediators for the acne inflammation.

4. Hormones: Hormonal factors regulate the function of sebaceous glands and sebum production.

a) *Testosterone metabolites* (dihydrotestosterone, dihydroepiandrosterone, androstendion, and androstendiol) increase the rate of mitosis and epithelial proliferation of sebaceous gland acini with following enhanced lipid synthesis (= sebum overproduction).

b) *Estrogens:* suppress sebum production through the hypophysis by decreasing circulating testosterone (= negative feedback mechanism). A direct sebum suppressive effect on the sebaceous glands is also presumed.

Forms of acne particularly influenced by hormonal factors are: Acne neonatorum, acne infantum, premenstrual acne, acne postpubertalis gestagenes, female androgenetic acne, and postadolescent acne of the back. Hormonal assays, however, often fail to find significant alterations of the circulating androgens.

5. Heredity: Genetic factors are strongly involved in acne development and influence the clinical pattern, the distribution of the lesions, and the duration of the susceptibility.

Familial incidence is increased in the severe forms of acne (e. g., acne conglobata). There are rare forms of very severe acne with XYY-syndrome. The mode of inheritance is assumed to be multi-factorial.

6. Immunological factors involved in acne inflammation are:

a) T-lymphocytes are sensitized against cell membrane antigens of Propionibacterium acnes (in acne with severe inflammation).

b) Lesions of follicle walls cause lymphokines of T-lymphocytes to attract activated macrophages which in turn, destroy the follicle and the peri-follicular tissue.

c) A genetic determination of the cell-mediated immune response is assumed.

The modern therapy of acne

1. *Retinoic acid:* Topical medicament with an exfoliating effect.
2. *Benzoyl peroxide:* Topical medicament with a bacteriostatic and an exfoliating effect.
3. *Antibiotics (tetracyclines, erythromycin, clindamycin etc.):* Topical and systemic medicaments with a bacteriostatic effect and a direct inhibition of extracellular lipases which decreases free fatty acids and cholesterol, and increases triglycerides.
4. *13-cis-retinoic-acid:* Oral medicament with a sebum suppressive and exfoliating effect.
5. *Antiandrogens:* Oral medicaments.

   Cyproterone acetate has a central inhibitory effect on androgen production in the ovaries and the adrenal cortex and blocks androgen-dependent sebum overproduction in the sebaceous glands.

Dermatological indications for anti-androgens are: Acne vulgaris, seborrhoea oleosa, sebocystomatosis, apokrine miliaria, androgenic alopecia, hirsutism and virilism.

The clearest indication for an anti-androgenic treatment is the association of acne with hirsutism in a women with an abnormal increase in ovarian or adrenal androgen production (polycystic ovaries, adrenogenital syndrome, etc.), or with an increase of androgens which is not otherwise treatable.

Materials and methods

Diane-35® is a combination preparation. 1 dragee contains 2 mg cyproterone acetate and 35 μg ethinyl estradiol. *Neo-Eunomin®* is a two-phase-preparation. 11 tablets contain 1 mg chlormadinone acetate combined with 50 μg ethinyl estradiol and 11 tablets contain 2 mg chlormadinone acetate combined with 50 μg ethinyl estradiol. A multi-center randomized double-blind clinical study with these two preparations in female patients with mild to severe acne vulgaris was performed to compare the effectivity of Diane-35® and Neo-Eunomin® in this disease. Patients accepted for the study were 18 to 35 years of age. Contraindications for hormone treatment were excluded and all patients gave their informed consent. The study is still ongoing. Here we present the results in 50 patients who participated in this randomized study over 6 treatment cycles. Twenty-one patients were treated with Diane-35®, 29 with Neo-Eunomin®. The mean age in both groups was approximately the same. The *clinical features of acne* (comedones, papules, pustules, nodules and cysts) were counted and photographed before study begin, after 3, and after 6 cycles. Also body weight, blood pressure, number of hair washes, and side effects were recorded (fig. 1).

- Clinical features of acne
  - Comedos
  - Papules
  - Pustules
  - Nodules
  - Cysts
- Number of hair washes
- Body weight
- Blood pressure
- Side effects

Fig. 1 Parameter

During the first three cycles local treatment with benzoyl peroxide was allowed, if found necessary. A statistical evaluation was not possible because of the small number of patients.

Results

Figures 2 and 3 show the *total number of facial acne lesions* 3 and 6 cycles after begin of treatment with Diane-35® or Neo-Eunomin® in those patients without

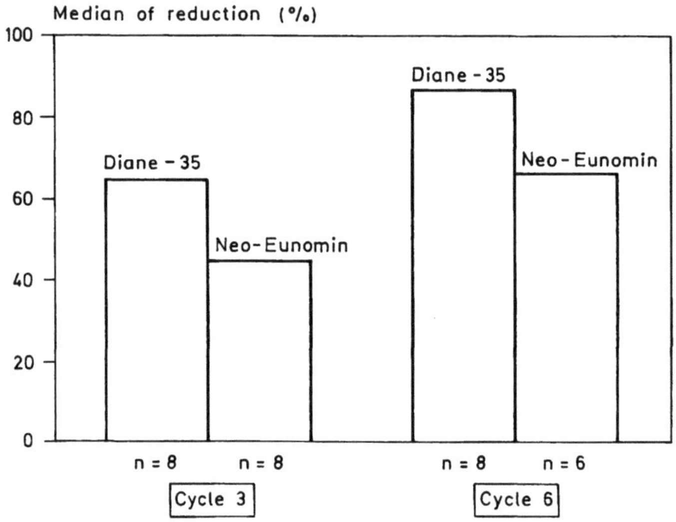

Fig. 2 Total number of facial acne lesions without BPO-treatment

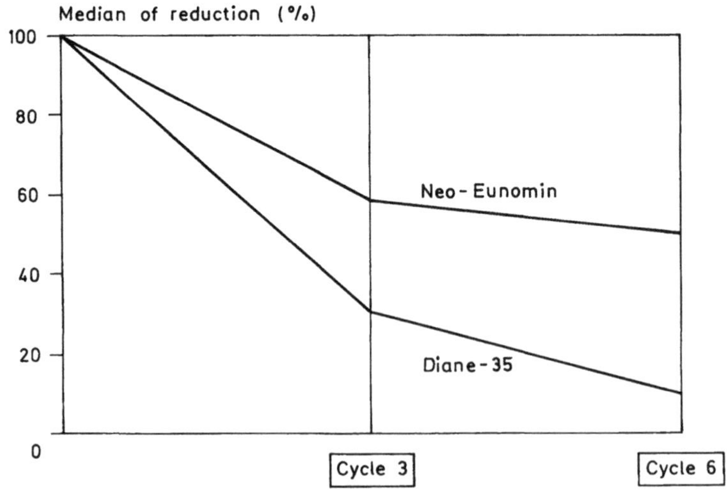

Fig. 3 Total number of facial acne lesions without BPO-treatment

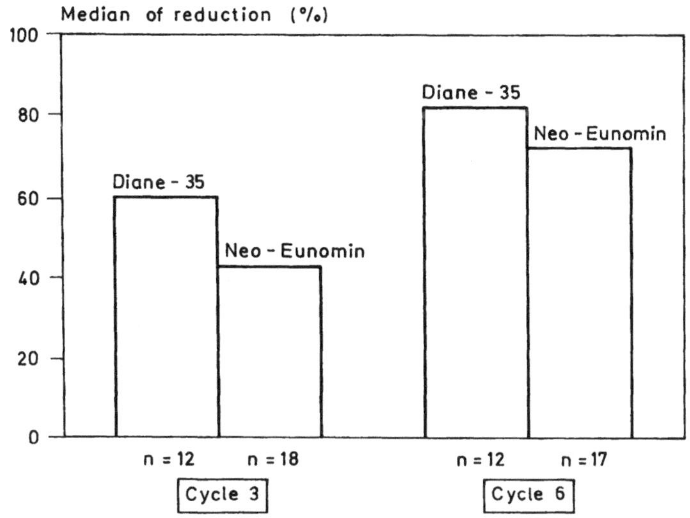

Fig. 4 Total number of facial acne lesions with BPO-treatment

additional benzoyl peroxide treatment during the first 3 cycles. In spite of the small number of patients, the reduction in all facial lesions after 3 cycles of treatment under both preparations is noticeable. The reduction with Diane-35® was more distinct, 68%, than with Neo-Eunomin®, 46%.

Facial lesions continued to subside during the entire 6 cycle treatment period (Diane-35®: 94%, Neo-Eunomin®: 72%).

Additional treatment with benzoyl peroxide did not seem to have a noticeable advantage over Diane-35® alone or Neo-Eunomin® alone (see fig. 4 and 5), but

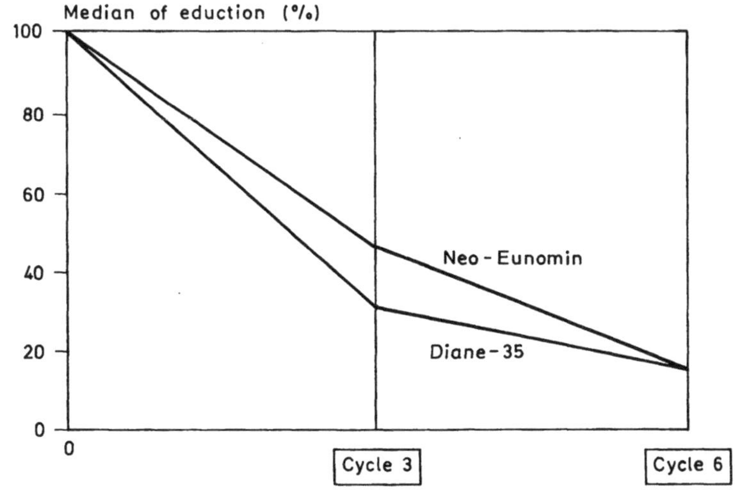

Fig. 5 Total number of facial acne lesions with BPO-treatment

the small number of cases should be remembered. Figures 4 and 5 demonstrate that during the first 3 cycles there was a marked decrease in acne lesions, which was more pronounced under Diane-35®. The reduction of acne lesions continued during the next 3 cycles, but not as rapidly as during the first 3 cycles.

The *overall-assessment* by the investigators of treatment with Diane-35® or Neo-Eunomin® alone showed, that Diane-35® was highly effective and better than Neo-Eunomin® for the treatment of acne vulgaris.

Body weight: Body weight remained unchanged during treatment with both preparations (fig. 6).

Fig. 6 Body weight

	Before treatment	3. cycle	6. cycle
Diane-35®	65,5 kg	65,3 kg	65,0 kg
Neo-Eunomin®	61,6 kg	62,5 kg	60,7 kg

Blood pressure: Blood pressure was not influenced (figs 7, 8, 9, 10).

Hair washes: The number of hair washes, which seemd to be influenced more by habitude than by necessity remained unchanged.

Figures 11 a—c show a 26-year-old patient before, after the 3 and after the 6 cycle treatment period with Diane-35®.

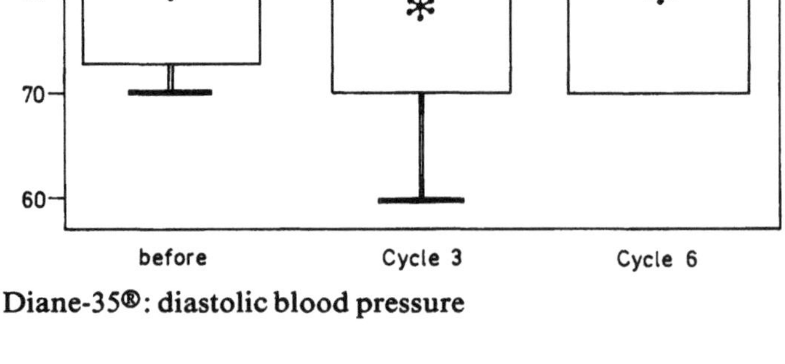

Fig. 7 Diane-35®: diastolic blood pressure

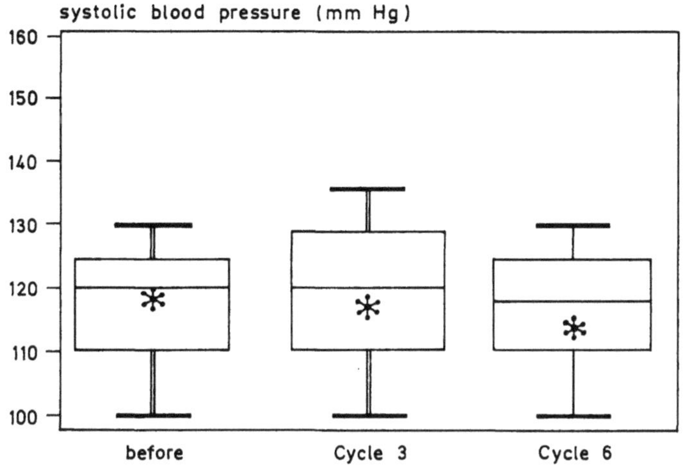

Fig. 8 Diane-35®: systolic blood pressure

Side effects

Breast tension and dizziness was observed more often under Neo-Eunomin® than under Diane-35® (fig. 12). This is probably at least partly due to the higher content of estrogen in Neo-Eunomin®. Other reportable side effects were not observed.

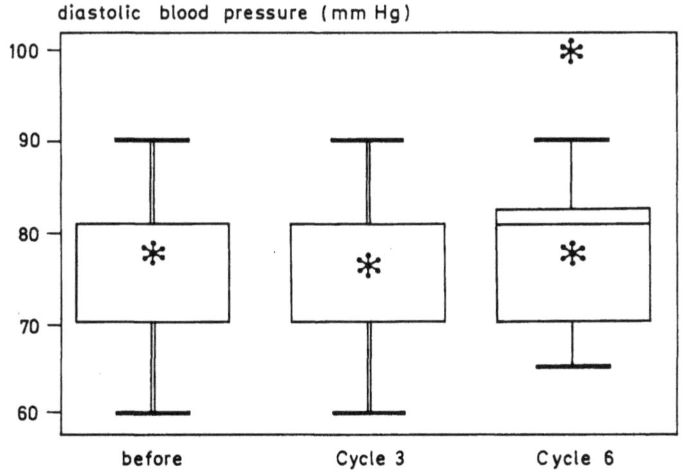

Fig. 9 Neo-Eunomin®: diastolic blood pressure

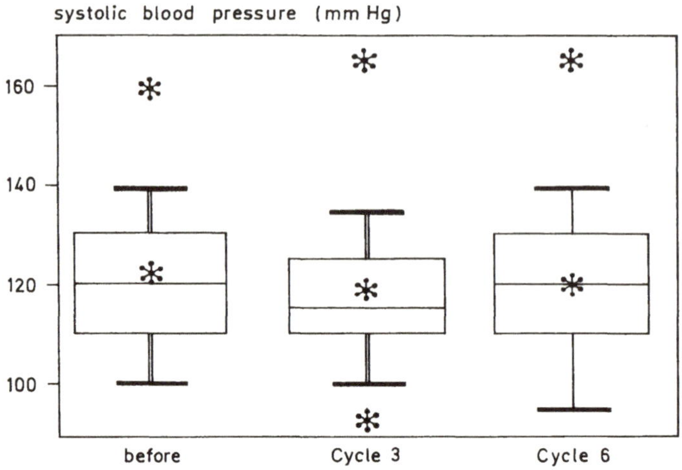

Fig. 10 Neo-Eunomin®: systolic blood pressure

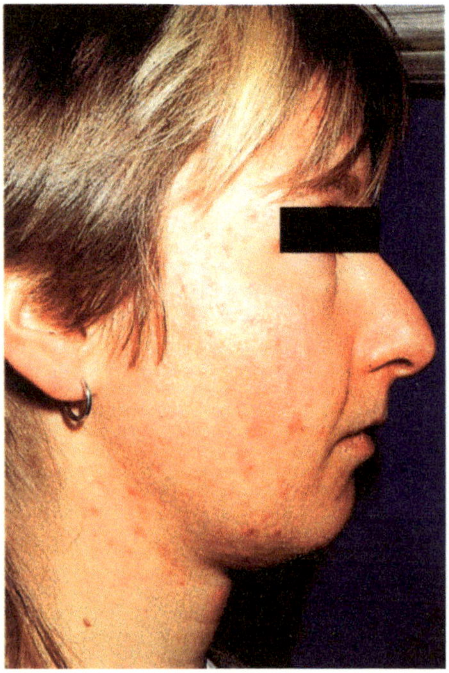

Fig. 11a

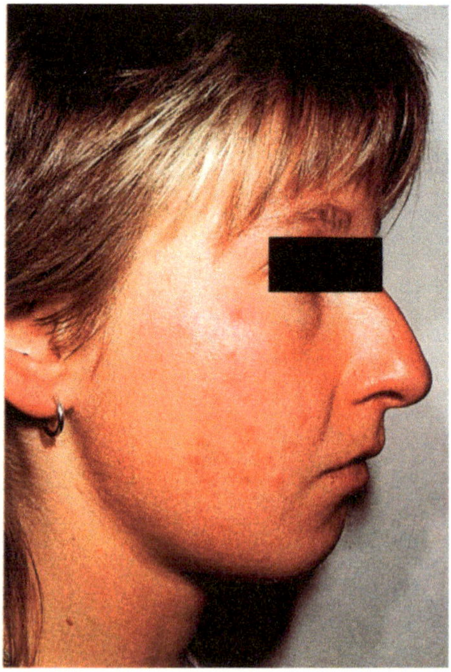

Fig. 11b

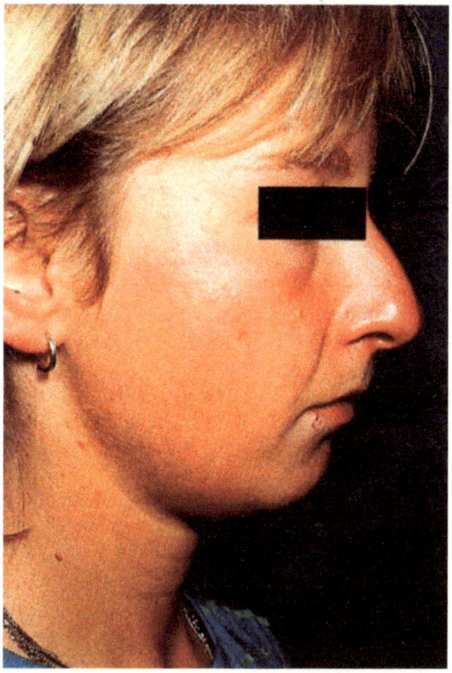

Fig. 11c

Fig. 11a–c A 26-year-old patient before (11a), after 3 cycles (11b) and after 6 cycles (11c) of treatment with Diane-35®.

Fig. 12 Side effects

	Diane-35®			Neo-Eunomin®		
	Before treatment	3. cycle	6. cycle	Before treatment	3. cycle	6. cycle
Breast tension	4.8%	9.5%	0	6.9%	10.3%	17.4%
Dizziness	0	0	0	3.5%	6.9%	4.4%
Nervousness	19.1%	4.8%	5.0%	6.9%	13.8%	4.4%
Depression	0	0	0	6.9%	6.9%	0

Conclusions

1. Hormone preparations with an antiandrogenic component can be effective in the management of acne vulgaris.
2. The prolonged trial of Diane-35® and Neo-Eunomin®, two new preparations with an antiandrogenic effect, showed that both preparations were effective in acne vulgaris.

3. The overall assessment of the preliminary study suggests that Diane-35® is superior to Neo-Eunomin®.
4. Additional topical treatment with benzoyl peroxide does not seem to offer an additional therapeutic effect in the first three cycles.
5. The side effects noted during 6 cycles treatment were tolerable.

References

[1] Plewig, G., A. M. Kligman: Acne: Morphogenesis and Treatment. Springer, Berlin 1975.
[2] Rook, A. et al.: Textbook of Dermatology. 4th ed. Blackwell, Oxford 1986.

A double blind comparative study of tetracycline and Diane®, alone and in combination in the treatment of acne

R. Greenwood, L. Brummitt, B. Burke, W. J. Cunliffe

Introduction

Acne is a chronic inflammatory disorder of the pilosebaceous unit. There are 4 important processes in acne. These are:

1. An increase in sebum production and alteration in its composition
2. Duct occlusion
3. Microbial colonisation, the most important being by Propionibacterium acnes
4. Host inflammatory response.

Diane® (50 μg ethinyl estradiol + 2 mg cyproterone acetate) affects acne by a mechanism different from that of tetracycline. Diane® reduces sebum excretion rate [1], while tetracycline affects the function of Propionibacterium acnes [2] and probably the host inflammatory mechanisms. As cyproterone acetate is both an antiandrogen and also a progestogen, it can be combined with ethinyl estradiol in order to provide contraceptive cover comparable to conventional combined oral contraceptives.

The aim of this study was to investigate how Diane® compared with tetracycline in the treatment of acne. Furthermore, since a combination treatment of Diane® and tetracycline may be seen as being superior to a single treatment, this too was investigated. Thus women who had already taken antibiotics for their acne were chosen for the double-blind randomized study. Clinical evaluation was performed by acne grading and lesion counts. In addition since ethinyl estradiol—cyproterone acetate and antibiotic treatment influence different etiological factors of acne the effect on sebum excretion and surface bacteria was assessed.

Materials

92 women aged 16—30 years with acne who had been referred from their general practitioners were recruited. Most patients had received low-dose anti-

biotic treatment previously. Patients were randomly allocated to one of 3 treatment groups. The treatment duration was six months.

Group 1 received Diane® (50 μg ethinyl estradiol and 2 mg cyproterone acetate) for 21 days out of 28 plus tetracycline 500 mg twice daily continuously (combination treatment).

Group 2 received Diane® (50 μg ethinyl estradiol and 2 mg cyproterone acetate) for 21 days out of 28 plus placebo tetracycline twice daily continuously.

Group 3 received placebo Diane® for 21 days out of 28 plus tetracycline 500 mg twice daily continuously.

Irrespective of whether the patients received placebo or active tetracycline they were told to take the antibiotic half an hour before meals with a sip of water to maximise absorption [3]. No topical treatment was given.

Patients were assessed at admission and after two, four and six months with a final post-treatment assessment two months later. Each patient was observed clinically by the same observer throughout the study. Clinical evaluation com-

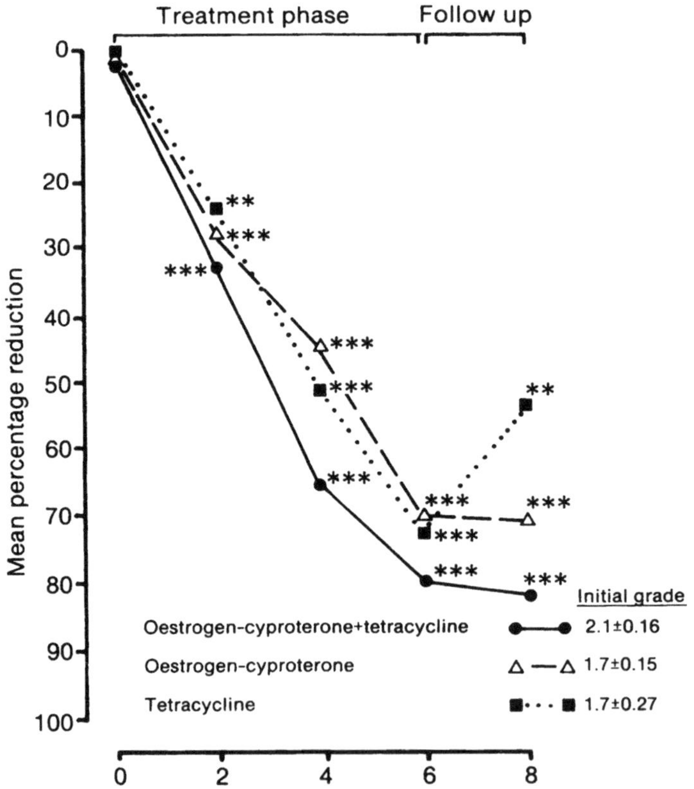

Fig 1

Fig. 1 Effect of three treatments on facial grade. Values indicate original acne score in arbitrary units. Compared with baseline: $^{**}p < 0.01$; $^{***}p < 0.001$.

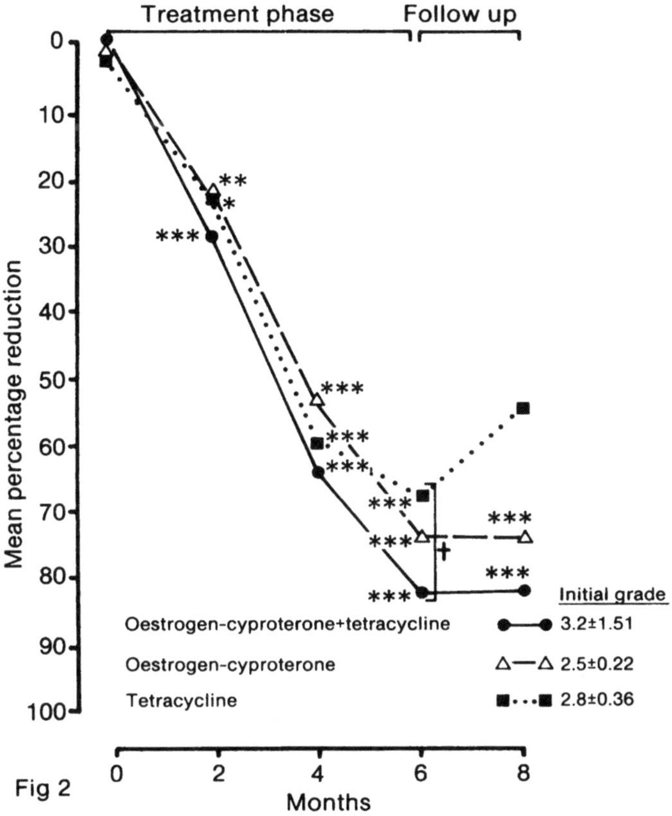

Fig 2

Fig. 2 Effect of three treatments on total grade. Values indicate original acne score in arbitrary units. Compared with baseline: $^{**}p<0.01$; $^{***}p<0.001$; $+p<0.025$.

prised of grading and counting of lesions [4]. The sebum excretion rate was measured at each visit by the gravimetric technique [5, 6]. Micro-organisms on the surface of the right cheek of 57 patients (22 in group 1, 18 in group 2, 17 in group 3) were sampled using the scrub technique of Williamson and Kligman [7].

Results

An error in the randomisation resulted in unequal numbers of patients per group. This difference, however, was not statistically significant and had no biasing effect on the results.

As can be seen from figures 1 and 2, all three treatment groups showed a gradual improvement in facial and total acne grade which was significant at all points compared with baseline. This overall improvement was reflected in a

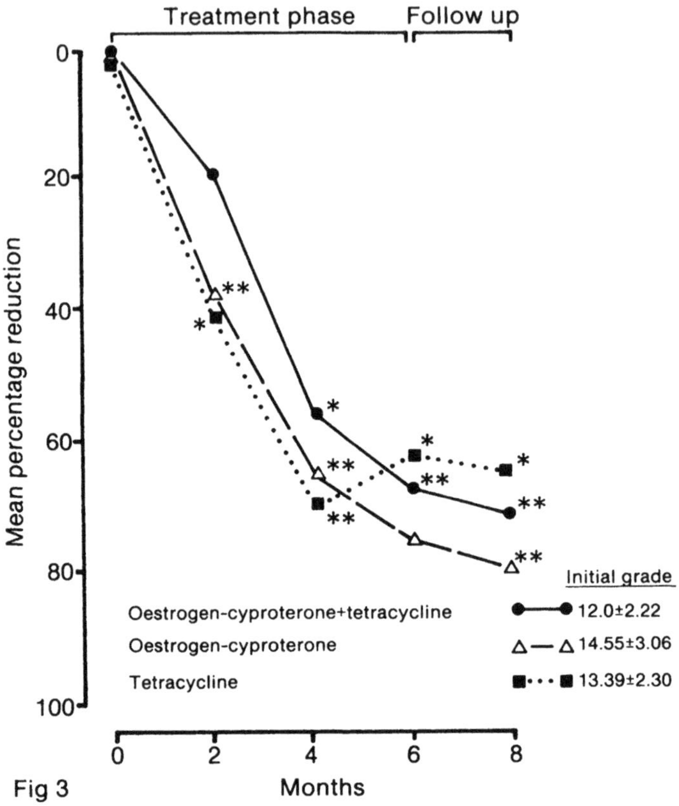

Fig 3

Fig. 3 Effect of three treatments on non-inflamed lesions. Compared with baseline: $^{*}p<0.05$; $^{**}p<0.01$.

significant reduction in non-inflamed and inflamed lesions (figs 3 and 4). At the end of six months the improvement in lesion counts varied between 51% and 80% (figs 3 and 4). The combination treatment (Diane® plus tetracycline) showed an 82% improvement in the total acne grade which was significantly better ($p < 0.025$) than that of the tetracycline group (fig. 2). Furthermore, a significant reduction in inflamed lesions between the same two groups was demonstrated at six months (fig. 4; $p < 0.001$). Diane® alone was not significantly different from either of the other two treatments.

Figure 5 shows the effect of the 3 treatments on sebum excretion rate. A significant reduction in sebum excretion rate was observed in both the Diane® and combination treatment groups throughout the study. The suppression of sebum excretion rate in the Diane® group was significantly greater than that seen in the combination treatment group at two months ($p < 0.05$). In the Diane® group, maximum suppression of 26.9% was seen at four months; in the combination treatment group a maximum suppression of 23.7% was seen at six months.

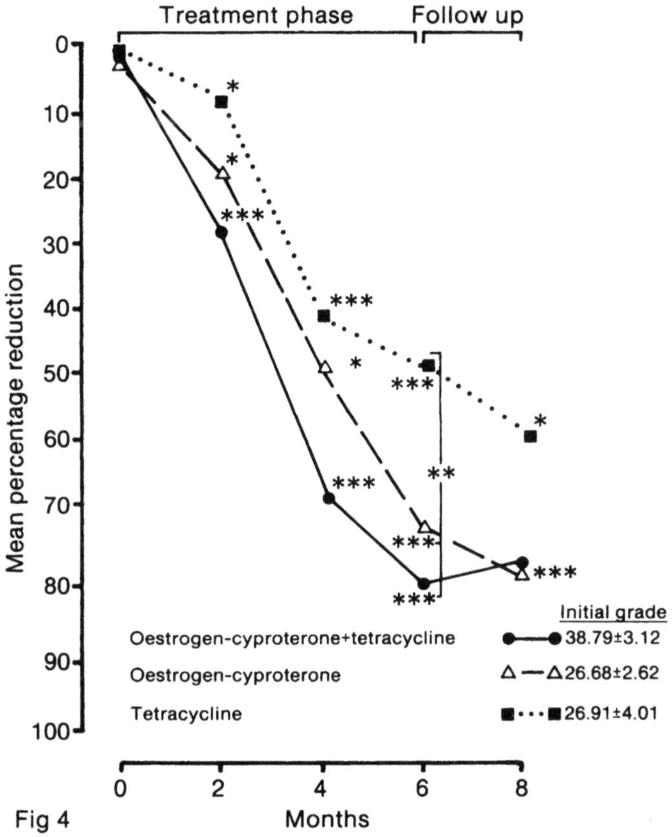

Fig. 4 Effect of three treatments on inflamed lesions. Compared with baseline: *$p<0.05$; **$p<0.01$; ***$p<0.001$.

The tetracycline group showed an increase in sebum excretion rate of about 7—13%. However, this was only significant at the two months assessment ($p<0.05$).

No significant reduction in the density of micrococcaceae on cheek skin was produced by any of the treatment groups. However, both tetracycline regimens achieved a significant reduction in counts of propionibacteria of the order of 1 log cycle, but the reduction was not significantly different between the two treatments.

When possible, patients were assessed at a two month post-treatment visit. A total of 50 patients attended; the breakdown was as follows:

Group 1 (Diane® plus tetracycline)—20 out of the 25 patients (80%)

Group 2 (Diane® plus placebo tetracycline)—14 out of the 21 patients (67%)

Group 3 (Diane placebo + tetracycline)—9 out of the 16 patients (56%).

No change was demonstrated in counts of inflamed and non-inflamed le-

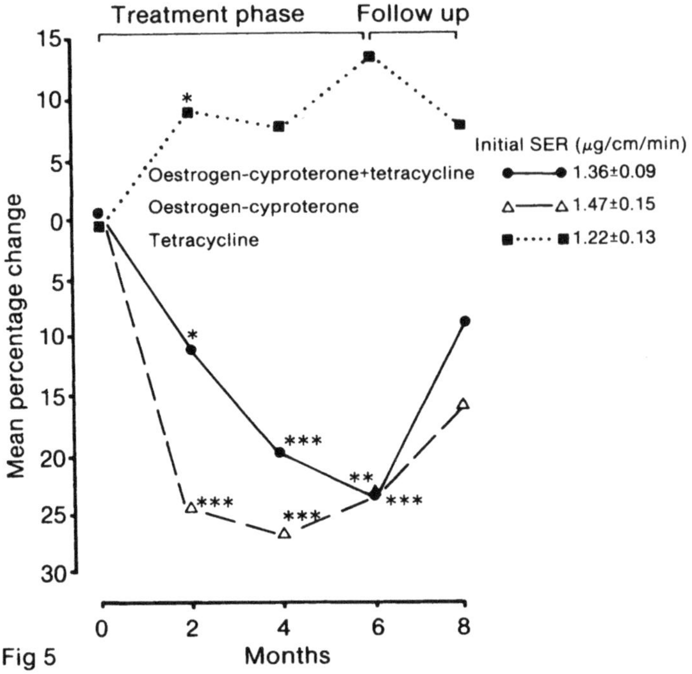

Fig. 5 Effect of three treatments on sebum excretion rate (SER). Compared with baseline: *$p<0.05$; **$p<0.01$; ***$p<0.001$.

sions. In the hormonal treatment groups the overall improvement in acne grade was maintained, but in the tetracycline group a relapse of acne occurred (fig. 1). Intergroup analyses showed that the antibiotic treatment group fared significantly less well than patients given the combined regimen ($p < 0.005$); improvement in facial acne grade was better maintained by both the combined treatment ($p < 0.001$) and the Diane® treatment ($p < 0.025$). Sebum excretion rate showed a return towards pre-treatment values after withdrawal of therapy in all groups (fig. 5).

Drop-outs and side-effects

A total of 30 patients withdrew from the study; the drop-outs were equally distributed per treatment group (tab. 1).
A variety of reasons were given for dropping out with the commonest being lack of compliance (11 patients). Seven patients withdrew due to the time-consuming nature of the measurement of sebum excretion rate. Side effects were common but usually minor. One patient taking Diane® developed mild, but de-

Table 1 Reasons for discontinuation of treatment

	Diane + Tetracycline	Diane alone	Tetracycline alone
Lack of compliance	4	2	5
Lack of efficacy	2	–	1
Wished to become pregnant	1	–	2
Sebum excretion rate: measurements too time consuming	1	5	1
Side effects:			
Chest pain	1	–	–
Headaches	1	–	–
Menstrual irregularity	1	–	–
Breast tenderness	1	–	–
Increased blood pressure	–	1	–
Dysmenorrhoea	–	1	–
Total	12	9	9

finite, hypertension which necessitated withdrawal; her blood pressure, however, returned to normal two months after stopping the drug. There was a small but significant weight gain in both Diane® treatment groups.

Discussion

Results from this study confirm those of previous studies [8, 9] showing that both Diane® alone and tetracycline alone administered over a 6 month period are effective treatments for acne. A significant improvement, as assessed by total and facial acne grades, was seen and maintained at 2, 4 and 6 months in both the Diane® and tetracycline groups. Spot counts suggested that a steady rate of improvement occurred between 4 and 6 months for all treatments. There was, however, a discrepancy between acne grade and lesion counts which may be explained by the fact that inflamed acne lesions show various intensities of inflamation [3]. This study, however, did not distinguish between the more active and less active inflamed lesions.

There have been no studies to investigate whether a combination of Diane® and tetracycline produces a greater benefit than either therapy alone. Both drugs affect acne by different mechanisms. Diane® reduces the sebum excretion rate [1], while antibiotics affect the function of Propionibacterium acnes [2] and probably the host inflammatory mechanism. It therefore seemed possible that Diane® and tetracycline may act synergistically. However, the results of this study did not support this hypothesis: there appears to be limited clinical benefit in this treatment combination.

Unexpectedly, the tetracycline treatment group showed an increase in sebum excretion rate up to a maximum of 13% which was significant at 2 months ($p < 0.05$). Other studies have failed to show an effect of antibiotics on sebum excretion rate [10]. The findings from this study, however, are unlikely to be due to a technical error since the patients started the treatments at different points in time and other concurrent studies carried out in the department did not produce any unusual results. It has been suggested that benzoyl peroxide, another antimicrobial agent, may affect sebum outflow [12] by reducing ductal cornification [11]. Since tetracycline also reduces non-inflamed lesions, an effect on sebum outflow may explain the increase in sebum excretion.

Tetracycline, by increasing the sebum outflow and thus sebum excretion rate, may attenuate the sebosuppressive action of Diane®. Alternatively, tetracycline, by affecting the gut bacterial flora, may reduce the enterohepatic recirculation of orally administered steroids [13]. This, in turn, may reduce the amounts of cyproterone acetate and/or ethinyl estradiol acting on the sebaceous gland. These two suggestions may explain why the effect of the combination treatment on sebum excretion rate seen at 2 months was not as great as the effect of Diane® alone ($p < 0.05$).

The mechanism by which Diane® suppresses sebum is unclear. There is no evidence as to whether it is the ethinyl estradiol or the cyproterone acetate which reduces the sebum excretion rate. Ethinyl estradiol alone in a dose of 60 μg has been shown to reduce the sebum excretion rate by 20% [14]. Oral contraceptives containing 50 μg ethinyl estradiol will reduce the rate by 34% [15] and might, therefore, be expected to ameliorate acne to a similar extent as Diane®. Cyproterone acetate given to men in a daily dose of 25 mg reduces the sebum excretion rate by 17% [16]. Cyproterone acetate without estrogen has not been given to women with an intact uterus because of its strong progestogenic action, which would probably produce menstrual irregularities. It seems unlikely that 2 mg cyproterone acetate is able to reduce sebum excretion by the amounts seen in our study. However, it appears that the combination of ethinyl estradiol with cyproterone acetate does have some benefit by suppressing sebum. Nevertheless, suppression of the sebum excretion rate by 25% is unlikely to explain the entire clinical benefits of the hormone treatment. There is indirect evidence that ductal cornification is controlled by hormones [12], and as Diane® significantly reduces non-inflamed lesions it is likely that it reduces ductal cornification. Whether this is a direct or indirect effect is uncertain. This study showed that although both tetracycline treatments significantly reduced the counts of propionibacteria, Diane® alone produced no effect. Thus an indirect effect of Diane® on bacteria in reducing comedogenesis seems unlikely.

Apart from the study by Greenwood et al. [9], only a few clinical or laboratory studies have reported follow-up assessments after discontinuation of treatment. It is known that, except for isotretinoin [17, 18], improvement in acne is inadequately maintained after cessation of therapy. Despite the short, only 2 months post-treatment follow-up period of this study, assessment of total and facial acne grades indicated that both the hormonal treatment groups were better than tetracycline alone in maintaining the improvement in acne.

Side effects were reported in all groups and, although responsible for some withdrawals, they were not a serious problem. The side effects did not differ significantly among the 3 treatment groups and the effects reported were those commonly associated with hormone treatments or antibiotics. The drop-out rates were also similar in the 3 groups.

We consider Diane® to be at least as effective as high-dose (1 g daily) tetracycline in the treatment of acne over a period of 6 months. However, 2 months after discontinuation of treatment acne relapsed at a greater rate in patients who had taken tetracycline compared to those who had taken Diane®. A combination of the two treatments showed no significant benefit over Diane® alone, but a greater improvement than tetracycline alone. It is unlikely that this complicated dual regime will be of any clinical value. Based on this study, we have shown an unquestionable benefit of Diane® which is similar to that of oral antibiotics. We suggest that it should be tried in the following groups of patients:

a) those whose oral contraception is jeopardised by antibiotic-induced diarrhoea, and
b) those whose acne has been improved by conventional treatment but shows no sign of further improvement after three to six months.

References

[1] Burton, J. L., U. Laschet, S. Shuster: Reduction of sebum excretion in man by the antiandrogen cyproterone acetate. Br. J. Dermatol. **89** (1973) 487—489.

[2] Webster, G. F., K. J. McGinley, J. J. Leyden: Inhibition of lipase production in Propionibacterium acnes by sub-minimal-inhibitory concentrations of tetracycline and erythromycin. Br. J. Dermatol. **104** (1981) 453—457.

[3] Kirby, W. M., C. E. Roberts, R. E. Burdilk: Comparison of two new tetracyclines with tetracycline and dimethylchoride tetracycline. In: Finland, M., E. M. Savage (eds.): Proceedings of first international conference on antimicrobial agents and chemotherapy, pp. 286—292. American Society for Microbiology, New York 1961.

[4] Burke, B. M., W. J. Cunliffe: The assessment of acne vulgaris. The Leeds technique. Br. J. Dermatol. **111** (1984) 83—92.

[5] Strauss, J. S., P. E. Pochi: The quantitative gravimetric determination of sebum production. J. Invest. Dermatol. **36** (1961) 293—298.

[6] Cunliffe, W. J., S. Shuster: The rate of sebum excretion in man. Br. J. Dermatol. **81** (1969) 697—704.

[7] Williamson, P., A. M. Kligman: A new method for the quantitive investigation of cutaneous bacteria. J. Invest. Dermatol. **45** (1965) 498—503.

[8] Mugglestone, C. J., E. L. Rhodes: The treatment of acne with an antiandrogen/oestrogen combination. Clin. Exp. Dermatol. **7** (1982) 593—598.

[9] Greenwood, R., B. Burke, W. J. Cunliffe: Evaluation of a therapeutic strategy for the treatment of acne vulgaris with conventional therapy. Br. J. Dermatol. **114** (1986) 353—358.
[10] Jones, D. H., W. J. Cunliffe, A. Loffler: A comparative study of 13-cis-retinoic acid and erythromycin in severe acne. In: Cunliffe, W. J., A. J. Miller (eds.): Retinoid therapy, pp. 293—301. Proceedings of international conference, London, May 1983. MTP Press, London 1984.
[11] Cunliffe, W. J., B. Dodman, R. Ead: Benzoyl peroxide in acne. Practitioner **220** (1978) 479—482.
[12] Holmes, R. L., M. Williams, W. J. Cunliffe: Pilo-sebaceous duct obstruction and acne. Br. J. Dermatol. **87** (1972) 327—332.
[13] Orme, M. C. E.: The clinical pharmacology of oral contraceptive steroids. Br. J. Clin. Pharmacol. **14** (1982) 31—42.
[14] Pochi, P. E., J. S. Strauss: Sebaceous gland suppression with ethinyl estradiol and diethylstilbestrol. Arch. Dermatol. **108** (1973) 210—214.
[15] Pye, R. J., G. Meyrick, M. J. Pye et al.: Effect on oral contraceptives on sebum excretion rate. Br. Med. J. **ii** (1977)1581—1582.
[16] Cormane, R. H., H. L. M. van der Meeren: Cyproterone acetate in the management of severe acne in males. Arch. Dermatol. Res. **271** (1981) 183—187.
[17] Jones, D. H., K. King, A. J. Miller et al.: A dose-response study by 13-cis-retinoic acid in acne vulgaris. Br. J. Dermatol. **108** (1983) 333—343.
[18] Peck, G. L., T. G. Olsen, F. W. Yoder et al.: Prolonged remissions of cystic and conglobate acne with 13-cis-retinoic acid. N. Engl. J. Med. **300** (1979) 329—333.

The comparative efficacy and safety of Diane-35® versus Diane-50® in the treatment of moderate to severe acne and seborrhea: preliminary results

P. Fugère, R. K. L. Percival-Smith, S. Lussier-Cacan, C. Tétrault, D. J. Farquhar

Introduction

Extensive multi-centre clinical trials with Diane® have amply demonstrated the effectiveness of the drug in the treatment of androgen-dependent acne, seborrhea and hirsutism [1, 3, 4, 5]. Many patients who had been refractory to conventional treatment, including tetracycline and vitamin A acid, have shown a positive and prompt response to Diane® [6].

The concept of employing an anti-androgen drug in the treatment of hormone-dependent acne is based on sound therapeutic principle. The safety of Diane® has also been demonstrated in thousands of women [1]. However, in order to improve even further the safety of contraceptive formulations, ever decreasing levels of ethinyl estradiol have been employed to minimize increases in serum lipid levels and any attendant risk of cardiovascular disease [2].

In accordance with this trend, a new lower-dose Diane® formulation has been prepared which contains just 0.035 mg ethinyl estradiol instead of 0.050 mg found in the original formulation.

In Canada, we were given the opportunity to compare the safety and efficacy of the lower-dose Diane-35® with that of Diane-50® in women with androgen-dependent skin conditions. When the study is completed, we will have data from 12 months of close clinical and laboratory observation. This presentation will provide the preliminary results of our multicentre trial, which was begun in late 1985 and is presently ongoing. The results here have been derived from two centres, Hôpital St-Luc in Montreal and the University of British Columbia in Vancouver. At the time of writing, women had completed up to 11 months of treatment, but numbers were only sufficient to analyze the first 6 months of treatment.

Methods and materials

Study design and drug administration

The study followed a double-blind design for parallel groups. At each centre, patients were randomly assigned to treatment with either Diane-35® (cyproterone acetate 2 mg and ethinyl estradiol 0.035 mg) or Diane-50® (cyproterone acetate 2 mg and ethinyl estradiol 0.050 mg). Neither the investigators nor the patients were aware of the identity of the test medications. The randomization code was maintained in the offices of the sponsor.

Diane-35® and Diane-50® were distributed in a special box containing 12 cycle packs. Each pack contained 21 identically appearing cream colored tablets. Treatment with both strengths of Diane® began with one tablet on day 5 of the normal cycle and continued in the same manner for the succeeding 21 days.

All previous systemic acne therapy had to be withdrawn within 6 weeks before start of treatment with Diane®. During the study, no concomitant anti-acne medication was permitted with the exception of mild cleansing agents. Likewise, no other concurrent medication was to be used by the patients while in the study.

Patient selection

Each patient enrolled in the study signed an approved informed consent form after the purpose and conditions of the trial had been carefully explained.

Patients considered for inclusion were women in good general health who presented with moderate to severe acne vulgaris. According to the rating scale used, moderate to severe acne was defined as the presence of comedones, papules and macules on at least half of the face. Many of the patients also suffered from concurrent seborrhea and/or mild hirsutism. The majority had been refractory to conventional topical or systemic therapy for acne.

The mean age of the patients in both treatment groups was 23 years (range: 17-35 years). None of the women was pregnant or contemplating pregnancy.

Prior to the start of the study, all the patients underwent a complete physical and laboratory examination (urinalysis, blood tests, SMA-12 and Pap Smear Class I or II) upon admission and every 6 months subsequently. The results were within the normal range at the start of the study.

Severe clinical criteria for inclusion were imposed. A patient exhibiting any one of the following conditions was automatically excluded: thromboembolic disorders, cerebral vascular disease, liver disease or liver dysfunction, known or suspected malignancy of the breast or genital tract, Cushing Syndrome, congenital adrenal hyperplasia, ovarian or adrenal tumors, known or suspected estrogen-dependent neoplasia, undiagnosed abnormal vaginal bleeding, ophthalmic vascular disease, myocardial infarction or classical migraine. Moreover, any patients receiving hormonal therapy for any reason were automatically excluded, as were those receiving a medication which might interfere with the activity of Diane® (such as cimetidine, dilaudid, phenobarbital).

Evaluations

As noted, each patient underwent thorough clinical, gynecological and laboratory examinations before entering the study. Throughout treatment with Diane®, the gynecologist regularly monitored body weight, blood pressure, cycle control and drug tolerance.

A dermatologist colleague performed all the pre-treatment evaluations of acne severity; he subsequently performed regular assessments of the patients response to Diane®. Specific ratings were employed for acne, seborrhea and hirsutism. In addition, a new 8-point rating scale was introduced with which the specific response of the three types of acne lesions (comedones, papules, macules) could be recorded. The dermatologist also provided a global rating of overall severity at each visit.

Metabolic studies were undertaken with the Montreal women in both treatment groups. During the third week of the cycle, blood samples were taken following a 2-hour fast. The plasma lipids and lipoprotein profiles (plasma total and lipoprotein VLDL-, LDL-, HDL2-, HDL3-cholesterol, triglycerides, apolipoproteins A and B) were determined every 3 cycles. Plasma total cholesterol, lipoprotein-cholesterol and triglycerides were measured by enzymatic methods on an autoanalyzer [6]. Lipoproteins were separated according to the Lipid Research Clinics protocol [6]. Lipid data are available for the first three cycles of therapy.

Statistics

The pretreatment demographic and gynecologic characteristics of both treatment groups were tested by the Student's t-test to confirm that the groups were well matched. Results of the acne rating scales and the gynecological factors indicating cycle control were submitted to an analysis of variance for a two factor experiment. Results for plasma lipids were analyzed before and after every 3 cycles using a Student's t-test. For all statistical analyses, the minimum level of significance was established at 5%.

Results

Patients

A total of 45 women entered the study, 23 at the Montreal centre and 22 at the Vancouver centre. The two geographic groups were found to be statistically comparable with respect to all the demographic and gynecological variables considered (age, height, weight, smoking/drinking habits, number of births or abortions in the history). All the women who entered the study are described in table 1 according to the treatment group to which they were randomly assigned. Following randomization, the two treatment groups were also found to be well matched.

At the time of cutoff, when the preliminary results had to be assembled for this presentation, a total of 9 patients (6 in the Diane-35® group and 3 in the Diane-50® group) had spent insufficient time in the study (≤2 cycles) to be included in the calculations. Three other patients, 2 in the Diane-35® group and 1 in the Diane-50® group, were withdrawn prior to establishing therapy with Diane® because of the appearance and possible interference from an unrelated concurrent disease. Two patients in the Diane-35® group discontinued the drug because of adverse effects during the second cycle. One of the patients complained of pain in her legs and the other of irritability, moodiness and increased appetite.

Table 1 Demographic characteristics of the patient sample

Variable	Mean (Range)	
	Diane-35 (N = 25)	Diane-50 (N = 20)
Age (years)	23.2 (18– 32)	23.7 (17 – 35)*
Height (cm)	161.9 (128–177.5)	160.3 (130 –175)*
Weight (kg)	62.1 (46– 88.8)	56.6 (42.3– 68.6)*
Race (N)		
– Caucasian	23	19
– Negro	1	0
– Asian	1	0
– Oriental	0	1
Smokers (N)		
Yes	3	4
No	22	16
Alcoholic (N)		
Yes	0	0
No	25	20
Age at menarche (years)	12.6 (9–15)	12.3 (10–17)*
Number of births	3	6
Number of abortions	2	3

* Between-group differences not significant by Student t-test

Thus, a total of 15 patients in the Diane-35® group and 16 patients in the Diane-50® group received Diane® therapy for a minimum of 4 cycles and were thus considered suitable for analysis. These patients were analyzed statistically from the baseline through the sixth cycle. Following the sixth cycle, numbers were insufficient to permit statistical evaluation.

Acne, seborrhea, hirsutism

Table 2 presents the comparative ratings for acne, seborrhea and hirsutism with the two strengths of Diane®.

At the start of treatment, the two groups showed similar characteristics. Moderate to severe facial acne was the dominant clinical feature, but acne of the neck and back as well as mild to moderate seborrhea and hirsutism were also present.

The women in the two treatment groups showed progressive improvement over time, which became apparent as early as the second cycle. Significant improvement in facial acne was recorded in the fourth cycle with Diane-35®, but not until the sixth cycle with Diane-50®, as compared to the baseline value. Although the anti-acne effect of Diane-35® appeared to be more rapid, there was no significant difference between treatments during any of the cycles.

A similar pattern was evident in the results for seborrhea. Both drugs produced improvement and, once again, Diane-35® was found to have a more

Table 2 Evaluations for acne, seborrhea and hirsutism: Diane-35 versus Diane-50

Variable	Mean Scores Reported over Six Cycles[a]							
	Diane-35				Diane-50			
	Cycle 0 (Pre-Rx)	2	4	6	0 (Pre-Rx)	2	4	6
ACNE								
Face	2.4	2.1	1.6**	1.8**	2.5	2.1	2.3	2.0**
Neck	1.8	1.5	1.4	1.4	1.6	1.4	1.5	1.3
Back	2.0	1.5	1.3	1.7	2.1	1.9	1.7	1.3
SEBORRHEA								
Greasy skin	1.9	1.5	1.3	1.6	2.0	1.6	1.6	1.4
Greasy hair	1.9	1.5	1.0*	1.5*	2.0	1.8	1.6	1.3*
Scale formation	1.4	1.1	1.1	1.2	1.1	1.2	1.1	1.1
HIRSUTISM								
Face	2.1	1.8	2.0	1.6	1.5	1.6	1.5	1.3
Chest	1.4	1.2	1.4	1.2	1.3	1.1	1.3	1.0
Legs	2.0	1.8	2.0	1.7	1.9	1.8	1.7	1.5

* $p<0.05$ versus baseline   ** $p<0.01$ versus baseline

a Scoring: 1 – not present
2 – mild
3 – severe

rapid onset (in cycle 4) than Diane-50®, which produced a significant response in cycle 6. This trend reached significance in the category of greasy hair, whereas the responses were not found to be significant in ratings for greasy skin and scale formation.

Hirsutism was, on average, a mild clinical symptom at the outset of the study and, although improvement took place, it was too gradual to establish any significant pattern.

Comedones, papules, macules and overall severity

In order to increase the sensitivity of the evaluations for acne, a new expanded 9-point scale was employed (see tab. 3). This rating scale, based on very specific clinical criteria, allowed us to record monthly changes with considerable precision. Likewise, the global evaluation for overall severity was based on a similar, expanded 8-point scale.

As illustrated in table 3, both formulations of Diane® provided significant improvement in all 3 types of acne lesions over time ($p < 0.01$). Diane-35® was associated with significant improvement versus the baseline in the ratings for comedones and papules starting with the second cycle. The significant change in macule lesions did not occur before the fourth cycle. In addition, the ratings for papules and macules showed further significant improvement with Diane-35® between cycles 2 and 4. With Diane-50®, a significant improvement

Table 3 Evaluations of comedones, papules, macules and overall severity: Diane-35 versus Diane-50

Variable	Mean Scores Reported over Six Cycles[a]							
	Diane-35				Diane-50			
	Cycle 0 (Pre-Rx)	2	4	6	0 (Pre-Rx)	2	4	6
Comedones	3.3	2.0*	1.3*+	1.3*	3.7	2.3*	2.5*	2.3*
Papules	4.0	2.3*	0.7*	1.7*	4.3	2.2*	2.6*	2.2
Macules	2.8	2.0	0.8*++	1.1*	3.6	1.4*	3.0	1.4*
Overall Severity	4.8	2.7*	0.9*+	1.4*	4.7	2.8*	3.0*	2.4*

* $p < 0.01$ versus baseline + Favors Diane-35 ($p < 0.05$) ++ Favors Diane-35 ($p < 0.01$)

a Scoring for comedones, papules and macules:
0 = Few isolated lesions permitted
1 = Few easily recognizable lesions
2 = Greater than grade 1; most of the face is clear
3–4 = More lesions; more facial involvement
5 = About half the face involved
6–7 = More than half the face involved
8 = Most of the face involved
9 = Entire face covered with lesions

Scoring for overall severity:
0 = Need not be perfect; scattered lesions
2 = No big or prominent lesions; few pustules
4 = Red lesions and significant inflammation; worthy of treatment
6 = Multiple comedones and pustules
8 = Conglobata, sinus or cystic type acne extending form face to neck and chin

as compared to pretreatment values was observed for all lesions in all cycles except for macules in cycle 4, when a temporary but significant worsening occurred.

In clinical terms, patients began the study with scores ranging from 2 to a maximum of 6—7 in the three categories of lesions. Thus, they characteristically presented with easily recognizable lesions covering approximately half of the face. Following 6 months of treatment with Diane®, only 3 patients had a score above 4, but none above 5. All 3 patients were in the Diane-50® group.

By the end of the fourth and sixth cycles, comedones, papules and macules had been virtually eradicated in 7 of the Diane-35® patients and 3 of the Diane-50® patients (scores of 0—1). This represents approximately one-third of the total number of women treated. Thus, the trend favoring Diane-35® remained consistent for all types of observations and was again reflected in the ratings for overall severity.

At admission to the study, ratings for overall severity ranged from 4—8 in both treatment groups (2 patients in each group had the maximum score of 8). Both Diane® formulations provided significant improvement in these ratings in each cycle as compared to pretreatment values, but with Diane-35®, additional significant change took place in cycles 4 and 6 versus cycle 2. The response with Diane-35® in the fourth cycle was also significantly better than that with Diane-50® ($p < 0.05$).

Cycle control

Throughout the study, the investigators monitored the patients regularly in order to determine the influence of Diane®, if any, on the cycle.

Length of cycle: the average length of the cycle at the baseline was 27 to 28 days in both groups. Good cycle control was maintained throughout the duration of the study with virtually no variation.

Duration of menstruation: good cycle control was also reflected in the uniformity of the length of the menstrual periods. In both treatment groups, menstruation was maintained for an average of 4.7 or 4.8 days from cycle 4 on.

Amount of flow: the majority of patients reported a normal flow at the baseline and throughout the study. Four women who began the study with an excessive flow (2 in the Diane-35® group and 2 in the Diane-50® group) reported a normalization in the amount of flow beginning at the end of the second cycle and continuing to the end of the study. Three patients in the Diane-50® group and one in the Diane-35® group reported a normal flow at the start of the study, but an increased amount of flow subsequently.

Amenorrhea: amenorrhea was not reported by any patient in the Diane-50® group at any time in the study. Three patients in the Diane-35® group reported being amenorrheic for a single cycle only (1 patient in cycle 4 and 2 in cycle 10).

Spotting: this clinical sign also occurred randomly with no apparent pattern. In the Diane-35® group, 1 patient reported spotting during cycles 6 and 8. Two other patients reported single episodes of spotting during cycles 4 and 8, respectively. In the Diane-50® group, 2 patients experienced single episodes of spotting in cycles 2 and 4, respectively.

Breakthrough bleeding: In the Diane-50® group, there was no incidence of breakthrough bleeding. In the Diane-35® group, 1 woman had experienced breakthrough bleeding prior to the institution of Diane® and up to the end of the second cycle; thereafter, she reported no further episodes. Three other patients each reported one isolated incidence of breakthrough bleeding in cycles 2 (1 patient) and 3 (2 patients).

Dysmenorrhea: prior to Diane® therapy, most patients had slight dysmenorrhea and 6 reported severe discomfort. In both treatment groups, the frequency and severity of dysmenorrhea decreased over time, although the trend was not statistically significant. After the fourth cycle, none of the women in either group experienced severe dysmenorrhea.

Tolerance

Both formulations of Diane® were well tolerated. Seven patients taking Diane-35® and 5 taking Diane-50® (or nearly 40% of the total) experienced no adverse effects at all. Table 4 charts the incidence of adverse effects with both treatments over the course of the study. It is clear that most of the adverse effects occurred in the first 2 cycles after Diane® was instituted. Thereafter, adverse effects were infrequent. As noted earlier, only 2 patients, both in the Diane-35® group, discontinued Diane® because of adverse effects.

Referring again to table 4, it can be seen that breast tension was the most common complaint (9 patients), of these, 2 were in the Diane-35® group and 7 were in the Diane-50® group. Nevertheless, none of the women complained of severe discomfort and the symptom usually did not persist beyond the second cycle.

Headache occurred in a total of 7 women. In one patient taking Diane-35®, migraine headache persisted on and off throughout the study; in 2 patients on Diane-50®, severe headaches were confined to the first treatment cycle. Four patients taking Diane-50® also complained of dizziness.

Gastrointestinal disturbances (nausea, vomiting, loss of appetite) occurred

Table 4 Summary of adverse effects with Diane-35 and Diane-50

Adverse Effect	Total No. Patients Reporting	No. Patients per Cycle						
		Cycle 1	2	3	4	5	6	8–11
DIANE-35								
NIL	7							
Breast tension	2	2	1					
Headache	3	1*	3	1	1*	1		1*
Nausea	2	2	1					
Vomiting	1	1						
Loss of appetite	1	1	1					
Sensitivity	1		1	1				
Agressiveness	2	1	2	1				
Nervousness	1		1	1				
DIANE-50								
NIL	5							
Breast tension	7	6	6	1	1		1	
Headache	4	3**	2		1	1	1	
Nausea	6	3	5	1	1	1	1	
Vomiting	3	2	1					
Dizziness	4	2	3					
Nervousness	1	1	1					
Edema	1		1					
Depression	1		1	1	1	1	1	
Varicose complaints	1			1	1	1	1	

* severe ** symptom severe in 2 of the 3 patients

occasionally early in therapy, but in only one patient (taking Diane-50®) did nausea persist past the second cycle.

Mood changes, such as nervousness, sensitivity, depression and aggression, were reported by a total of 4 patients in the Diane-35® group and by 2 patients in the Diane-50® group. One of the latter felt depressed throughout the study, but in her case there were extenuating circumstances unrelated to the treatment.

Body weight was monitored regularly during the study. There were no significant changes in body weight with either formulation. The mean body weights showed a slight tendency to increase in both groups, however, by only 5 or 6%.

Blood pressure also remained stable throughout the study. Neither systolic nor diastolic pressure showed any increasing or decreasing trends.

Lipid profile

Total plasma and lipoprotein lipids were measured prior to and after every third cycle in 17 of the Montreal women (7 in the Diane-35® group and 10 in the Diane-50® group).

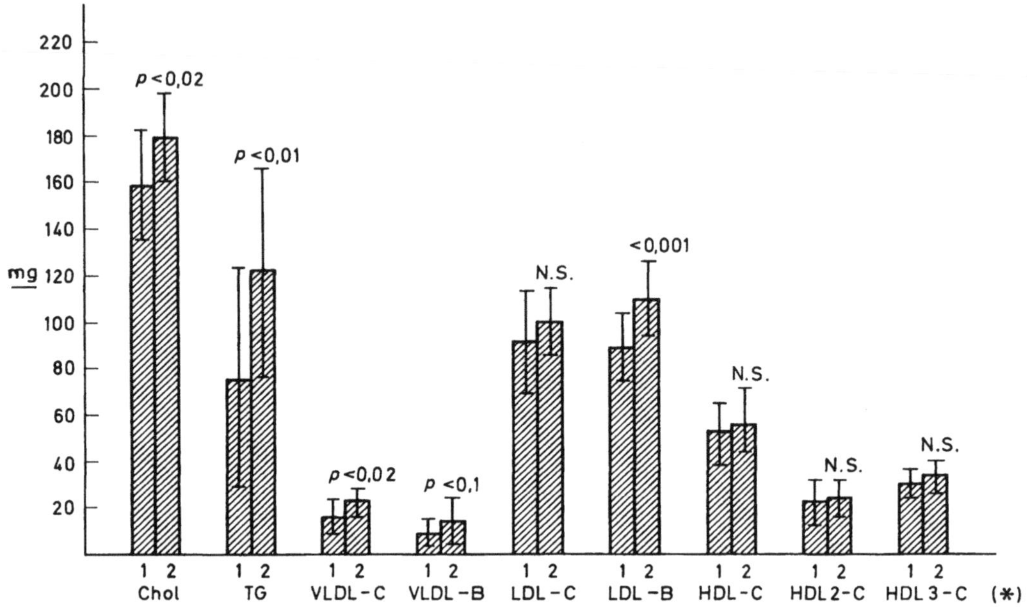

Fig. 1 Change in lipid profile with Diane-35® and Diane-50® (combined group of 17 patients) from baseline through fourth cycle
Chol: cholesterol
TG: triglycerides
VLDL-C: very low density lipoprotein-cholesterol
VLDL-B: very low density lipoprotein-apo B
HDL-C: high density lipoprotein-cholesterol

Cholesterol and triglycerides showed a tendency to increase in both treatment groups, but the increase was significant only for triglycerides in the Diane-50® group ($p < 0.01$). Because the patient numbers were small, values for all 17 patients were pooled. Calculations using the larger sample revealed significant increases with time in both cholesterol and triglycerides (see fig. 1).

Lipoproteins (VLDL, LDL, HDL, Cholesterol) also showed a tendency to increase over time in both treatment groups, but the changes did not reach significance in the individual treatment groups. After pooling the patients into one group, significant increases were observed for VLDL-C ($p < 0.02$) and LDL-apo B ($p < 0.001$). As figure 1 illustrates, these significant changes correspond to small numerical changes demonstrating that a larger patient sample will be required before a final interpretation can be made.

It is worthwhile noting, however, that despite the increases in the individual lipoprotein entities, there were no significant changes in the ratio of low to high density lipids, LDL-C/HDL-C, since both fractions increase similarly.

Discussion

Diane®, with its antiandrogen component, has widened the therapeutic scope for physicians and has provided an opportunity for gynecologists and dermatologists to collaborate for the distinct benefit of women with symptoms of androgenisation. In Canada, we have been highly satisfied with the very positive early results of this study. The patients have also shown a willing acceptance of the drug.

The effectiveness of both formulations of Diane® in treating acne and seborrhea was apparent within the first 2 months of treatment and was significant within 4 to 6 months. This time frame agrees closely with observations of other investigators [3, 4, 7].

The low-dose formulation of Diane® was just as active as the higher dose; in fact, there was some indication that Diane-35® was superior to Diane-50® in terms of the time of onset of the clinical effect and the magnitude of the effect. For example, acne lesions tended to recede gradually with Diane-50® over time whereas improvement with Diane-35® appeared to occur in larger month-to-month increments.

In terms of the proportion of patients showing clinical improvement in their acne condition, 6 patients receiving Diane-50® and 2 patients receiving Diane-35® remained refractory over the first 4 to 6 months of treatment. Thus, one may consider that the overall success rate was approximately 86% with Diane-35® and 60% with Diane-50®. The value for Diane-35® is in line with results published earlier concerning Diane-50® [3, 4], but for Diane-50® there was a lower rate of success in this study. The reason for this is not clear.

On the basis of the preliminary results, then, we can conclude that the therapeutic effect of Diane® is in no way diminished by reducing the level of ethinyl estradiol. On the contrary, there may be a therapeutic advantage associated with Diane-35®. This, however, remains conjecture until more data have been collected.

In both treatment groups, cycle control was excellent. In fact, we believe that all aspects of cycle control are superior with Diane® than with other contraceptives currently in use. In addition, blood pressure remained stable and mean body weights increased only slightly. Gaspard et al. [3] also reported a mean weight gain of 2.4 kg over 6 months of treatment, which agrees closely with our findings. Adverse effects, when they occurred, were usually mild and most were confined to the first 2 months of therapy.

Again, in agreement with Gaspard [3], we found that mean lipid levels increased slightly over the first 6 months of treatment. Although the numbers were too small to draw any conclusions, there was some indication that the relative rise in lipid levels was smaller with Diane-35®. If this observation is eventually confirmed in a larger sample of women over 12 months or more, Diane-35® will represent a definite advantage in terms of clinical safety. It should be emphasized, however, that although significant increases were found in serum lipid and lipoprotein levels, the values still remained well within their normal ranges.

References

[1] Data on File, Schering AG, Berlin/Bergkamen, West Germany.

[2] Fotherby, F.: Oral contraceptives, lipids and cardiovascular disease. Contraception **32** (1985) 367—394.

[3] Gaspard, U. J., M. A. Romus, M. Soyeur-Broux et al.: Clinical, endocrinological and metabolic evaluation of women treated for acne by a combination of cyproterone acetate and ethinylestradiol (Diane®). In: Vokaer, R., D. Fanta (eds.): Combined antiandrogen-estrogen therapy in dermatology, pp. 75—94. Excerpta Medica, Amsterdam, Oxford, Princeton 1981.

[4] Keller, P. J.: Clinical experiences with antiandrogenic oral contraceptives. In: Vokaer, R., D. Fanta (eds.): Combined antiandrogen-estrogen therapy in dermatology, pp. 95—100. Excerpta Medica, Amsterdam, Oxford, Princeton 1981.

[5] Khodjasteh, Z., G. Copinschi, C. Lejeune-Lenain et al.: Hormonal profile acne before and during six months' Diane® administration. In: Vokaer, R., D. Fanta (eds.): Combined antiandrogen-estrogen therapy in dermatology, pp. 101—108. Excerpta Medica, Amsterdam, Oxford, Princeton 1981.

[6] Lussier-Cacan, S. et al.: apo E allele frequency in primary endogenous hypertriglyceridemia (IV) with and without hyperapobetalipoproteinemia. Arterial Sclerosis **5** (1985) 639—643.

[7] Thulliez, M.: Diane®: le point de vue d'un dermatologue belge. In: Vokaer, R., D. Fanta (eds.): Combined antiandrogen-estrogen therapy in dermatology, pp. 71—73. Excerpta Medica, Amsterdam, Oxford, Princeton 1981.

Results of an extended open phase III study with Diane-35®

S. Aydinlik

Introduction

Diane®, an antiandrogen-estrogen combination, has proved to be highly effective in the treatment of signs of androgenization in women [1, 4, 5, 6, 9, 10, 12, 13, 14]. Diane® contains 2 mg cyproterone acetate and 0.050 mg ethinyl estradiol per single dose.

Since the lowest effective dose should always be administered, the reduction of the estrogen content of Diane® seemed desirable. In pursuit of this, and on the basis of dose-finding studies by Professor Haspels we developed Diane-35®. The two preparations differ only in the dosage of the estrogen component. Diane-35® contains 35 mcg ethinyl estradiol, that is, 15 mcg less than Diane®.

In order to find out whether Diane-35® is as effective as Diane® in the treatment of signs of androgenization in women and whether the new product causes fewer of the estrogen-related side effects which occasionally affected the tolerance to Diane®, a multi-centre, double-blind, comparative study was conducted for 9 cycles with the two preparations from 1982—1984. Recruited to the study were 425 women with signs of androgenization such as acne, seborrhoea, or mild hirsutism [2, 11].

The results of this study, which covers 3250 cycles, show that the therapeutic effects of Diane-35® and Diane® hardly differ and that the positive results

Table 1 Healing and improvement of all acne cases (severe and mild)

	Cycle 3		Cycle 9	
	Diane	Diane-35	Diane	Diane-35
Face	41.7%	51.9%	89.6%	91.5%
Neck	42.5%	45.3%	91.6%	89.9%
Back	52.7%	45.9%	92.2%	93.5%

Referred to the total number of women

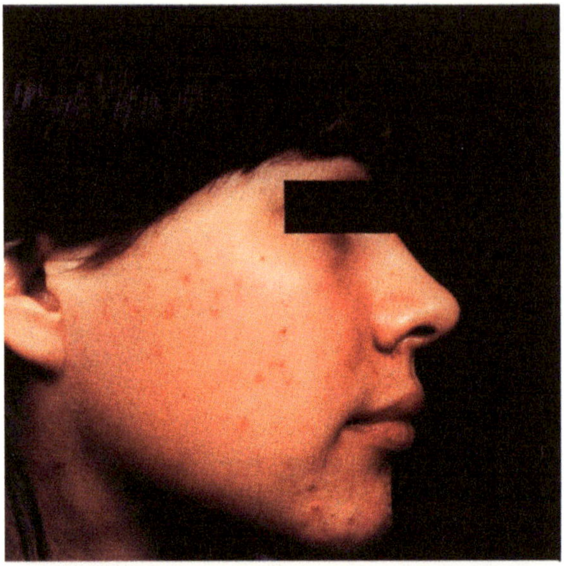

Fig. 1a

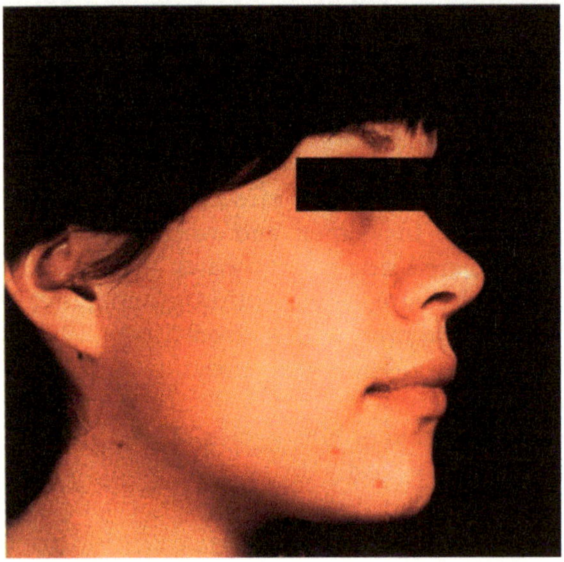

Fig. 1b

Fig. 1 Moderately severe juvenile acne
a) before treatment
b) after 4-months treatment with Diane-35®

of the treatment were recognisable more quickly with Diane-35® than with Diane® (fig. 1). This very important finding was confirmed by other investigators in Canada, Holland, and Sweden. The healing and improvement rates for all acne cases are summarized in table 1.

Table 2 Side effects

	Diane-35	Diane
Breast tension	20.2%	28.0%
Edema	1.0%	2.4%
Varices	3.2%	5.3%
Vomiting	0.5%	3.4%
Dizziness	4.1%	5.8%

Referred to the total number of women

Although the healing and improvement rates in the 3rd cycle are better for Diane-35®, there are no significant differences between the two preparations. The results are similar for the treatment of seborrhoea. The estrogen-related side effects were less frequent under Diane-35® than under Diane® (tab. 2).

This difference is statistically significant ($p<0.05$) for some estrogen-dependent side effects such as breast tension and vomiting. A significant difference ($p<0.05$) for changes of weight in favor of Diane-35® is also recognisable throughout the trial period. At the end of the 9th cycle an increase in weight of more than 2 kg was observed in only 13.2% of the women on Diane-35®, while in women on Diane® the corresponding rate was 21.0%.

Diane® and Diane-35® produced very similar cycle control, although the rates of intermenstrual bleeding were slightly higher under Diane-35® than under Diane®.

Phase III study

The double-blind study was followed by an extensive open multi-centre, phase III study, the object of which was to gain a better idea of the favourable effect of Diane-35® in signs of androgenization and also to determine whether the preparation provides reliable contraception as well as its good cycle control and tolerance.

The study was commenced in 1984 in Germany, Austria, Holland, France, and Italy both in hospitals and among gynecologists and dermatologists with their own practices. The latest interim evaluation of this study already covers 10,653 cycles. A total of 875 women were recruited to the study, all of whom displayed the signs of androgenization mentioned-above and accepted the simultaneous contraceptive effect of the preparation.

802 women, or 91.7% of the total, received the preparation for 6 cycles; 611, or 69.8%, for 12 cycles; 223 for 18 cycles; and 64 women for more than 24 cycles. The study is scheduled to end next year. Although intake errors were ad-

mitted in 210 cycles, only one pregnancy occurred during the treatment period documented. This could be unequivocally attributed to patient error.

Cycle control

As in the double-blind study, the cycle pattern under Diane-35® was very similar to that under other modern estrogen-progestogen combinations (tab. 3).

Table 3 Intermenstrual bleeding rates in 10.215 cycles under Diane-35

Spotting	5.2%
Breakthrough bleeding	0.9%
Spotting and Breakthrough bleeding	0.4%

A comparison of correct and incorrect tablet taking shows, as expected, that the rates are much lower among correct tablet takers (tab. 4).

Table 4 Intermenstrual bleeding rates under Diane

	with intake errors (210 cycles)	without intake errors (10.005 cycles)
Spotting	20.0%	4.9%
Breakthrough bleeding	4.8%	0.8%
Spotting and Breakthrough bleeding	1.4%	0.3%

The anticipated withdrawal bleeding failed to occur in only 24 of 10,653 cycles under Diane-35®. This results in an amenorrhoea rate of 0.2%, which must be regarded as low.

Side effects

Side effects were documented in the last cycle before the start of treatment and after every treatment cycle. Calculation of the mean values for the percental incidence of side effects for the 24-month period of the study and comparison with the initial values produce the results given in table 5.

The highly favourable influence of the preparation on dysmenorrhoea is particularly striking. The rate of occurence of other side effects show significant changes compared to the initial values, although many side effects are, in fact, less serious under the treatment.

Although some of the women in the study have now completed 24 cycles of treatment, changes of weight have been rare. Body weight under Diane-35® re-

Table 5 Subjective and objective side effects

	Pre-treatment %	Cycle 1–24 %
Dysmenorrhoea		
light	21.1	9.5
severe	6.5	0.2
Headaches	6.8	4.3
migraineous type	1.3	0.2
Libido		
increased	0.2	0.4
decreased	2.6	2.2
Dizziness	2.3	0.9
Breast tenderness	8.9	5.5
Nervousness	8.9	3.7
Depressive moods	5.5	2.0
Chloasma	3.7	3.0
Edema	1.8	1.4
Varices	2.4	2.6

Calculated in terms of total number of treatment cycles

mained unaffected in 89.7% of the women in the 3rd cycle, in 86.5% in the 6th cycle and in 82.25% in the 12th cycle.

The long-term documentation of the blood pressure values indicates a favourable effect of Diane-35® on this parameter. In the 12th cycle of treatment, the systolic blood pressure was within the normal range in 97.5% of the women.

The influence of the preparation on the diastolic blood pressure values was particularly pleasing. Diastolic pressure reverted to the normal range in a surprisingly large number of women with high initial values of 90—105 mmHg. In the 12th cycle under Diane-35® the number of women with values below 90 mmHg was 96.5%. We must wait and see whether this interim result is confirmed in the final evaluation.

Therapeutic effect

The study was originally planned to be conducted in women with only mild to moderate signs of androgenization. However, women with severe symptoms were recruited in the trial: the facial acne group consists of 451 women with mild and 323 women with moderately severe to severe acne.

Table 6 shows the healing and improvement rates for all acne cases during the 12-month treatment period.

Table 6 Healing/improvement of all acne cases (mild and severe)

	Cycle 3	Cycle 6	Cycle 12
Face	36.2%	68.9%	90.5%
Neck	33.7%	71.5%	87.6%
Back	37.2%	69.2%	88.1%

The healing and improvement rates for severe and moderately severe acne are even more impressive (e.g., 98.5% in the 12th cycle for facial acne).

Good therapeutic results were also recorded in cases of mild facial hirsutism. Complete disappearance after 12 months of treatment was observed in 33.8% of these cases.

These results are similar to those from the double-blind study.

Comparative study

The results of a double-blind study carried out in Sweden demonstrated the superiority of Diane® and Diane-35® over Microgynon®, a contraceptive containing levonorgestrel. We obtained similar results in an open comparative study with a desogestrel-containing monophasic contraceptive, Marvelon® which was conducted in Finland.

It is a known fact that, because they reduce ovarian biosynthesis of androgens, oral contraceptives can exert a favourable effect on acne, which is why this comparison was conducted [3, 7, 8].

Composition of the trial preparations:

Diane-35®

2 mg cyproterone acetate

0.035 mg ethinyl estradiol per tablet

Marvelon®

0.150 mg desogestrel

0.030 mg ethinyl estradiol per tablet

The study lasted 9 months. A total of 162 women took the study preparations for 1,276 cycles: 84 women took Diane-35® for 658 cycles and 78 women took the reference preparation over 618 cycles.

Some of the results were very interesting: Cycle control was good under both preparations; however, spotting and breakthrough bleeding were recorded somewhat more frequently, but not significantly, under Marvelon® than under Diane-35® (tab. 7).

The influence of the two preparations on signs of androgenization was, of course, of particular interest. The healing and improvement rates for all acne cases were superior to those of Marvelon®. The difference was statistically

Table 7 Intermenstrual bleeding rates

	Diane-35®	Marvelon®
Treatment cycle	610	555
Spotting	2.5%	4.0%
Breakthrough bleeding	1.1%	2.8%
Spotting and Breakthrough bleeding	0.8%	0.8%

Expressed as percentage of total number of cycles

significant ($p < 0.05$) in cases of facial acne and also of greasy skin throughout the study (tab. 8).

Table 8 Healing and improvement of all cases of facial acne

	Diane-35®		Marvelon®	
	Cycle 3	Cycle 9	Cycle 3	Cycle 9
Facial acne	58.4%	80.7%	38.4%	63.3%

Referred to the total number of women

Table 9 Side effects

	Diane-35® Cycle 1–9 (%) (658 cycles)	Marvelon® Cycle 1–9 (%) (618 cycles)
Dysmenorrhoea		
slight	4.6	6.2
severe	0.5	0.9
Headaches	6.9	7.2
migraineous type	4.4	4.3
Libido		
increased	–	–
decreased	0.7	4.6*
Nervousness	3.1	7.6*
Depressive moods	3.5	7.1*
Breast tenderness	2.9	9.1*
Chloasma	–	–
Edema	4.3	4.3
Varices	0.5	1.5

Referred to the total number of cycles *$p < 0.05$

Differences were also observed between the side effects associated with the two preparations. Breast tension, nervousness, depression, varices, and reduced libido were recorded significantly more frequently under Marvelon® than under Diane-35® ($p < 0.05$) (tab. 9).

Conclusion

It is clear from all three studies that Diane-35® fulfills the requirements for optimal therapy for signs of androgenization in women.

At 35 mcg estrogen per single dose, it also meets the modern demand for the lowest possible dose of estrogen. The therapeutic results show that the estrogen-antiandrogen combination is superior to any other estrogen-progestogen therapy. The reduction of the estrogen dose in Diane-35® compared to the dose in the tried and tested preparation Diane® did not lead to any reduction of the therapeutic effect. On the contrary, there is even a tendency for an earlier onset of action. In addition, the potential for estrogen-related side effects appears to be lower under the new preparation.

References

[1] Aydinlik, S., U. Lachnit-Fixson: Diane – eine Gestagen-Östrogen-Kombination mit Antiandrogenwirkung. Med. Mschr. **31** (1977) 425—429.

[2] Aydinlik, S., U. Lachnit-Fixson: Östrogenreduzierter Ovulationshemmer zur Aknetherapie. Fortschr. d. Med., 27—28, pp. 547—551 (1986).

[3] Barfield, W. E.: Acne successfully treated by inhibition of ovulation. J. Amer. med. Ass. **201** (1967) 30.

[4] Carlborg, L., S. Rosengren: Antiandrogen Treatment of Women with Acne Tarda. Curr. Ther. Res. **31** (1982) 740—745.

[5] Fanta, D., W. H. F. Schneider, J. Spona et al.: Die Anwendung von Antiandrogenen in der Behandlung der Akne. Wien. klin. Wschr. **89** (1977) 622—627.

[6] Gaspard, U. J. et al.: Clinical, endocrinological and metabolic evaluation of women treated for acne by a combination of cyproterone acetate and ethinylestradiol (Diane®). In: R. Vokaer, D. Fanta (eds.): Combined antiandrogen-estrogen therapy in dermatology, Proceedings of the Diane Symposium, Brussels, Sept. 11, 1980, pp. 75—93. Exerpta Medica, Amsterdam 1981.

[7] Kümmel, J.: Beeinflussung der Akne vulgaris durch Ovulationshemmer. Med. Welt (Stuttgt.) **17** (1966) 138—140.

[8] Lachnit-Fixson, U., J. Kaufmann: Zur Beeinflussung von Androgenisierungserscheinungen. Doppelblindstudie eines cyproteronacetathaltigen Präparats (SHB 209 AB) gegen Neogynon®. Med. Klin. **72** (1977) 1922—1926.

[9] Ludwig, E., W. Meinhof, H. Zaun: Zur Therapie androgen-abhängiger Hauterscheinungen mit Cyproteronacetat-Östrogen-Kombinationen. Akt. Dermatl. **3** (1977) 201—209.

[10] Moltz, L., E. Kaiser: Mittelhochdosierte orale Cyproteronacetat-Therapie bei Frauen mit mittelgradig ausgeprägten Androgenisierungserscheinungen — Ergebnisse aus einer multizentrischen Doppelblind-Studie. Geburtsh. u. Frauenheilk. **44** (1984) 47—52.

[11] Neumann, F., S. Aydinlik, U. Lachnit-Fixson: The treatment of androgen-induced or mediated disorders of the skin with cyproterone acetate, In: N. Bruchovsky, A. Chapdelaine, F. Neumann (eds.): Regulation of Androgen Action. Proceedings of an Intl. Symposium, Montreal 1984, 109—113. Congressdruck R. Brückner, Berlin (West) 1985.

[12] Neumann, F., U. Lachnit-Fixson: Sexualhormone: Zielorgan Haut — Anwendungsmöglichkeiten von Antiandrogenen in der Dermatologie. Ärztl. Praxis **100** (1978) 346—347.

[13] Palatsi, R., P. Ylöstalo, A. Taipale: Treatment of acne with cyproterone acetate and ethinyl estradiol. Acta Dermatovener (Stockholm) **58** (1978) 449—454.

[14] Zaun, H.: Ovulationshemmer und Antiandrogene in dermatologischer Indikation. Fortschritte der praktischen Dermatologie und Venerologie. Band 9, herausg. von O. Braun-Falco u. H. H. Wolff, Springer, Berlin/Heidelberg 1979, 371—376.

Discussion

Samsioe: I take the opportunity as chairman to congratulate all speakers for the excellent presentation of their studies. I wish to stress that such investigations are very difficult to perform since there are seasonal changes in acne. In addition, one cannot recruit a control group and patient compliance may be bad. Furthermore, I would like to make some comments regarding the results of metabolic studies. The use of the ultracentrifuge method to determine the lipoprotein concentrations results in an underestimation of increases in HDL. In addition, results obtained by precipitation methods have to be interpreted with caution. This is due to the calculation methods used, which take into acount a certain distribution of triglycerides between the lipoproteins. This fraction may vary under the influence of estrogens and may, therefore, lead to erroneous results in the calculation, especially of LDL. Also, the differentiation between HDL_2 and HDL_3 can lead to erroneous results when the well-established dextran method is used. The reason for this is that triglyceride concentrations may influence the analysis and may result in an overestimation of HDL_2 by the precipitation method. The papers of the morning session have to be discussed bearing these considerations in mind.

The papers of the session "Metabolic and clinical aspects" are open for discussion.

Mrs. Schindler: The papers of Dr. Silfverstolpe and De Jacob combined seem to suggest that the results obtained are independent of the type of progestin used and are not influenced by the amount of ethinyl estradiol used. I wish to remind you that 20 and 50 μg ethinyl estradiol, resp., were used in the two studies.

Silfverstolpe: We found a difference in the serum VLDL concentration between the two groups of patients taking the 35 μg and 50 μg ethinyl estradiol combination. This difference was, however, not statistically significant because of the very small number of patients recruited.

Samsioe: I wish to use the privilege of the chairman to ask Mrs. Levinska (Burke) to expand on her observation that the application of Diane® alone and Diane® plus tetracycline does not result in any differences. Could tetracycline cause this phenomenon? This antibiotic was shown to reduce the enterohepatic circulation of hormones and may, therefore, have caused these results. Would you please comment on this?

Levinska (Burke): Yes, reduced SER in groups that were treated with Diane® plus tetracycline suggest the hypothesis that the enterohepatic circulation of steroids is reduced by tetracycline. Therefore, this explanation can also be used to interpret data presented by our group.

A dutch dermatologist: Yesterday, Dr. Ashton showed that the use of high dose cyproterone acetate resulted in a faster response rate than did low dose cyproterone acetate. In the studies presented today it seems as if Diane-35® results in a faster response rate than the use of Diane-50® in acne patients. Would the use of a higher dose of CPA added to that used in Diane-35® result in a further improvement in acne patients?

Gaspard: Data presented by our group clearly indicate that a combination containing 35 μg ethinyl estradiol plus 5 mg cyproterone acetate does not result in a faster response than observed by a 2 mg cyproterone acetate combination in acne patients and in patients suffering from seborrhea.

Falsetti: If I recall the data presented correctly the 5 mg CPA combination gave the same increase in SHBG as a 2 mg CPA combination. Could you then comment on the action of CPA?

Gaspard: If you recall my data, the increase in SHBG was three times over that of the baseline. The values stayed quite stable with time. The effects observed with the combination CPA plus ethinyl estradiol are quite different from those observed with the combination ethinyl estradiol plus 19-nortestosterone. In the combinations using 19-nortestosterone derivatives as progestins, a clear-cut blunting of SHBG serum levels by 19-nortestosterone derivatives can be observed. The antiestrogenic action of CPA is very small and the increase in SHBG is attributable to the effect of ethinyl estradiol alone, without a counteraction of a progestin component. This is very different from observations with 19-nortestosterone derivatives instead of CPA.

Schindler: It was shown that the combination of 2 mg CPA containing 35 μg ethinyl estradiol results in a faster response than the combination containing 50 μg ethinyl estradiol. But, the response rate of the 50 μg ethinyl estradiol combination becomes equal to that of the 35 μg ethinyl estradiol combination at later time such as 6 or 9 months. Does anyone have an explanation for this observation?

Lachnit: The faster response to Diane-35® may be at least partially explained by data presented by Prof. Spona. He showed that endogenous 17β-estradiol is suppressed to a smaller extent than registered with Diane-50® during the first 3 cycles. This may result in more favourable overall serum levels of estrogens and could, therefore, cause a more rapid response. I wish to draw your attention to studies performed by Prof. Breckwoldt many years ago. He compared the high-dose original Hammerstein scheme with the regular Diane®. He observed a similar phenomenon as that reported today. Response rates were faster in the beginning but leveled off at 12 months of therapy. These results are in favour of the notion of using the lowest possible dose of hormones.

Vermeulen: I wish to make a comment on the greater efficacy of Diane-35®. Observations in a small number of patients indicate that Diane-35® suppresses androstendione serum levels to a greater extent than does the Diane® containing 50 μg ethinyl estradiol. This difference in 5α-androstendione may explain the faster response rate to Diane-35®.

Samsioe: We feel that early response to therapy is of great importance in acne patients in order to obtain a high patient compliance. Therefore, a faster response rate with Diane-35® is of great importance. Are there any further questions?

Schindler: What were the contraceptive precautions in the group of patients who were on tetracycline only in Dr. Burke's study.

Levinska (Burke): The protocol of the study called for the use of other contraceptive precautions in all groups of patients.

Denvoers (Dutch dermatologist): The studies presented so far have shown that Diane-35® is superior to Diane® with respect to a faster onset of therapy results. Could you further improve these results by adding an additional dose of CPA to that used in Diane-35® for treating acne patients?

Lachnit: As you have seen, Diane-35® results in a fairly quick onset of therapy effects. There is no reason why one could not add 5 or 10 mg CPA to Diane-35® if one wishes. 10 mg CPA ist available in tablets. But, I would advise that it not be added during the whole cycle because of the great depot effect of CPA. Therefore, 5 or 10 mg CPA should be given from day 1 through 15 in order not to interfere with withdrawal bleeding.

Übachs: Could an increase of CPA over that used in Diane-35® improve the cure rate of hirsutism?

Lachnit: The 2 mg CPA dose in Diane-35® is high enough for mild facial hirsutism. But, in severe hirsutism the CPA dose should be increased.

Aydinlik: Facial hirsutism responds to Diane-35® treatment better than hirsutism at other localizations. We observed that Diane-35® resulted in elimination of facial hirsutism in 34% of patients. But, therapy results with Diane-35® for other localizations are not as good as those observed in facial hirsutism.

Nürnberger: I agree with you that Diane-35® is good enough for patients with facial hirsutism. You should treat patients with severe hirsutism with Diane-35® adding at least 10 mg CPA from day 1 through day 15.

Karger: We use 100 mg CPA in addition to Diane® for the treatment for severe hirsutism and acne. I wonder whether you can give any comments on this.

Lachnit: You have to add CPA to Diane® in patients with severe hirsutism and acne. I think Prof. Schindler can make further comments on that.

Schindler: There has been experience with Diane® for more than 10 years now and there is full agreement that one has to differentiate between the therapy of seborrhea, acne, and very mild forms of hirsutism and the treatment of severe hirsutism. In the first group of indications Diane-35® will suffice, but in severe forms of hirsutism 100 mg of CPA has to be added during the first part of the cycle, i.e., from day 1 through day 15. But I would not recommend using CPA in addition to an oral contraceptive containing a 19-nortestosterone derivative as the progestin component. I can recommend using 100 mg in a reversed sequential manner in combination with ethinyl estradiol. Once you get an onset of therapy effect you can slowly reduce this high CPA dose in order to arrive at a dose where a sustained therapy effect can be maintained.

Lachnit: This is a recommendation which we fully agree with. You can cut down on the dose of cyproterone acetate as soon as as full therapy effect is observed, i.e., after approximately 12 months, and continue to treat the patients with Diane-35®.

Spona: I refer to the presentation of data by Mrs. Aydinlik. She showed that Marvelon® and Diane-35® differ in their therapy results only in facial areas, whereas no differences in therapy effect could be registered in other localisations of hirsutism. Do you have any explanations for these results.

Aydinlik: At present we cannot offer any explanations for these differences.

Lachnit: If there are no further questions, I wish to thank, on behalf of Schering Italy and also Schering Berlin, the participants in this interesting meeting. I greatly appreciate the contributions by all speakers and the comments in the discussions. Many thanks also to Prof. Falsetti and to the President of the meeting, Prof. Schindler.

Closing remarks

U. Lachnit-Fixson

In conclusion I would like to summarize some of the important findings and statements of this conference:

1. There can be no doubt any more that cyproterone acetate-ethinyl estradiol preparations are highly effective in the treatment of signs of androgenization in women.
   With regard to acne treatment, they represent a valuable addition to the therapeutic armamentarium of the dermatologist.
2. The therapeutic effectiveness of the 2 mg cyproterone acetate combinations is not only due to the well-known suppression of androgen biosynthesis following inhibition of ovulation.
   Double-blind studies have clearly demonstrated a superior effect of these combinations in comparison to reference products containing progestogens without a partial antiandrogenic action.
3. In comparative trials it could be shown that Diane-35® exerts the same therapeutic efficacy as Diane-50®, even with a trend towards a somewhat earlier manifestation of the beneficial effect.
   So we can say that none of the therapeutic qualities has been sacrificed by decreasing the estrogen dosage.
   However, the incidence of estrogen-related side effects was significantly reduced which is important not only for better tolerance, but also for better patient compliance.
   Furthermore Diane-35® guarantees full contraceptive protection and its cycle control compares favorably with that of low-dose oral contraceptives containing derivatives of 19-nortestosterone.
4. Diane-35® has remarkably few adverse effects on metabolic and haemostatic parameters, thus taking into account aspects of medical safety. In fact, some of the observed changes—for instance in lipid metabolism—can be classified as rather beneficial.

Our workshop is approaching its end. We had two very interesting days, and I sincerely hope that you enjoyed the conference.

I want to thank all of you for your participation, in particular, of course, our President, Prof. Schindler, all the speakers for their presentations and all chairmen for their moderation.

List of first-mentioned contributors

Ashton, R. E., Dr., Royal Naval Hospital, Gosport-Hents, PO 12 2AA, Great Britain

Aydinlik, S., Clinical Endocrinology and Fertility Research, Schering AG, Müllerstraße 172—178, 1000 Berlin 65, Germany

Bruni, V., Prof. Dr., Clinica Ostetrica e Ginecologica della Università di Firenze, Policlinico Careggi, 50 134 Firenze, Italy

Carlborg, L., Dr., Department of Obstetrics & Gynecology, Länssjukhuset, Kvinnokliniken, 301 85 Halmstad, Sweden

De Cecco, L., Prof. Dr., 2nd Obstetrical Gynaecological Clinic, University of Genoa, Genoa, Italy

Ernst, E., Priv.-Doz. Dr., Klinik für Physikalische Medizin der Universität München, Ziemssenstraße 1, 8000 München 2, Germany

Falsetti, L., Prof. Dr., 1. Clinica Ostetrica e Ginecologica dell'Università Spedali Civili, 25 100 Brescia, Italy

Fedele, L., Prof. Dr., Istituto Ostetrico Ginecologico 'L. Mangiagalli' dell'Università di Milano, 20 122 Milano, Italy

Flamigni, C., Prof. Dr., Fisiopatologica della Riproduzione, Policlinico S. Orsola, 40 138 Bologna, Italy

Fugère, P., Dr., Hôpital Saint-Luc, Université de Montréal, 1058 rue Saint-Dénis, Montréal H2X 3J4, Quebec, Canada

Gaspard, U. J., Prof. Dr., Faculté de Médecine, Clinique gynécologique et obstétricale, Boulevard de la Constitution 81 (Bât. J15), 4020 Liège, Belgium

Greenwood, R., Dr., Dermatology Department, Leeds General Infirmary, Leeds, West Yorkshire, Great Britain

Haspels, A. A., Prof. Dr., Academisch Ziekenhuis Utrecht, Universiteitskliniek voor Obstetrie en Gynaecologie, Postbus 16250, 3511 GV Utrecht, Netherlands

Higgins, H. P., Dr., Departments of Dermatology, Leicester Royal Infirmary, Infirmary Square, Leicester LE 1 5WW, Great Britain

Hirvonen, E., Dr., Departments I and II of Obstetrics & Gynecology, University Central Hospital, Helsinki, Finland

Kaiser, E., Prof. Dr., Deutsche Klinik für Diagnostik, Fachbereich Gynäkologie/Gynäkologische Endokrinologie, Aukammallee 33, 6200 Wiesbaden 1, Germany

Lachnit-Fixson, U., Dr., Clinical Endocrinology and Fertility Research, Schering AG, Müllerstraße 172—178, 1000 Berlin 65, Germany

Neumann, F., Prof. Dr., Main Department Endocrine Pharmacology, Schering AG, Müllerstraße 172—178, 1000 Berlin 65, Germany

Nürnberger, F., Prof. Dr., Hautklinik und Poliklinik der Freien Universität Berlin im Rudolf-Virchow-Krankenhaus, Augustenburger Platz 1, 1000 Berlin 65, Germany

Rubens, R., Dr., Afdeling Endocrinologie — Hematologie, Stofwisselingsziekten, Akademisch Ziekenhuis, De Pintelaan 185, 9000 Gent, Belgium

Schindler, A. E., Prof. Dr., Direktor Zentrum für Frauenheilkunde, Universitätsklinikum Essen, Hufelandstraße 55, 4300 Essen 1, Germany

Silfverstolpe, G., Dr., University of Göteborg, Department of Obstetrics & Gynecology, Sahlgren's Hospital, 41345 Göteborg, Sweden

Spona, J., Prof. Dr., I. Universitäts-Frauenklinik, Spitalgasse 23, 1090 Wien, Austria

Zurth, Chr., Dr., Dept. Pharmacokinetics A, Schering AG, Müllerstraße 172—178, 1000 Berlin 65, Germany

Bei Fragen zur Produktsicherheit wenden Sie sich bitte an:
If you have any questions regarding product safety,
please contact:

Walter de Gruyter GmbH
Genthiner Straße 13
10785 Berlin
productsafety@degruyterbrill.com